Delinquency and Parental Pathology

A STUDY IN FORENSIC AND CLINICAL PSYCHOLOGY

DELINQUENCY AND PARENTAL PATHOLOGY

A Study in Forensic and Clinical Psychology

ROBERT G. ANDRY M.A., Ph.D., F.B.Ps.S., F.A.Ps.S.

*Senior Clinical Psychologist, St Thomas's Hospital
and Lecturer in Psychopathology, and Director-in-Charge of
The Diploma Course in Educational Rehabilitation of Young
People, Institute of Education, University of London*

Staples Press London

Granada Publishing Limited
First published in Great Britain 1960 by Methuen & Co Ltd
Revised edition published 1971 by Staples Press
3 Upper James Street London W1R 4BP

ISBN 0 286 62756 6
Printed in Great Britain by Fletcher & Son Ltd
Norwich and London

364.36

DEDICATED
TO MY FAMILY

CONTENTS

ACKNOWLEDGEMENTS

The writer wishes to express his sincere thanks to those who have helped him with this investigation.

He wishes to express particular gratitude to Professor Norval Morris, and Dr A. W. Meadows (respectively in the faculties of Law and Psychology of the University of Adelaide, Australia). Their friendship as well as skill and enthusiasm in criminology and that of Dr E. Cunningham-Dax, Dr H. K. B. Bailey, Dr Val Ashburne, the late Mr Justice J. Barry, and Mr E. Slattery, of Melbourne, have been constant sources of inspiration.

He is also very much indebted to various officials of the London County Council and in particular to Mr Childs, Mr Ainscow and Mr Wheeler, as well as to Mr Walters and Mr Clerk, and their respective staff. Equal gratitude is also expressed to the late Captain Harvey and his staff of an L.C.C. Remand Home and especially to Dr Peter Scott, Dr John Rich, Mr B. Lorraine, Mrs S. McConville and Dr C. H. Franks, formerly of the Maudsley Hospital.

Gratitude for statistical help and advice is also expressed to Mr L. T. Wilkins, Mr T. David and Mr W. Gleeson.

Very special thanks are due to Dr A. N. Oppenheim and Dr Elizabeth Nelson for their constant help and advice throughout an earlier stage of this study.

Dr Hilde Himmelweit of the London School of Economics has been of very great assistance. Also of great help in their encouragement have been Sir Cyril Burt, Professor Vernon, Professor Sprott and especially Professor Mace.

A very special mention must be reserved for the well-known Criminologist Dr Hermann Mannheim, without whose ever-ready council, patience and understanding this study could not have been carried through.

Finally, the author wishes to acknowledge his great debt to his colleague Gordon Coulson without whose masterly editing and criticism this book would never have appeared in its present form, and to the many children and parents without whose help this could never have been written.

LONDON, 1960   R. G. A.

ACKNOWLEDGEMENTS
to the Second Edition

The author, in reviewing the literature since the last decade, wishes to thank as much as ever before, Dr Hermann Mannheim, O.B.E.; his wife, Ann, for having acted as his editor, and Miss Caroline More and Miss Ann Fuller for typing the manuscript. Further, he wants to record his indebtedness to some who have either been of direct or indirect assistance in recent times; among these many should be singled out almost at random: Hugh Klare, C.B.E., the late Derek Morrell, Head of the Home Office Children's Department, Mrs Clare Winnicott, Professor Philip Vernon, Professor and Mrs Sheldon Glueck, Professor Leslie Wilkins, and Professor Norval Morris, as well as his colleagues, publisher and members of his family, especially his late father.

In reviewing some of the more recent literature of the last decade in this version (at the beginning and end of this book but not in the main text) the author is impressed with the fact that basically very little new research has emerged which has tended to upset his basic hypothesis, which suggests that fathers may have a special role to play in the aetiology of some delinquents.

LONDON, 1971   R.G.A.

FOREWORD

Scientific progress usually seems to take a zigzag course. Whether this can best be expressed in terms of Hegelian dialectics as thesis, anti-thesis, and synthesis or by any other general formula, it is probably true to say that most scientific theories are in the first instance framed in terms far too sweeping and uncompromising to remain unchallenged for any length of time. Other, often equally extreme, theories proclaiming the very opposite are likely to appear on the scene, soon in their turn to be replaced by a third view which tries to reconcile the first two and eventually becomes the starting point of a new dialect process. Sometimes such an antagonism takes the form of clashes between different scientific disciplines. The history of criminology, in particular, shows frequent changes from predominantly sociological to predominantly biological, psychological, or psychiatric interpretations of crime and criminals, and from the latter back to the original, though refined and modernized, sociological explanation. It also happens, however, that within the sphere of sociological or within that of psychological theories a similar zigzag course can be observed.

To the study of the part played by defective family relationships in the evolution of crime and especially juvenile delinquency these considerations apply with particular force. Here we are concerned with problems which can be approached with perhaps equal justification from all those widely differing viewpoints mentioned before. Here, too, we have witnessed profound changes in prevailing attitudes to certain specific phenomena, such as for example mental defect as a causal factor in delinquency, occurring within the boundaries of one discipline, psychology. To give but one illustration, to regard low intelligence as an important causative factor, as used to be the case fifty years ago, is now entirely out of fashion. Such changes are in no way surprising, nor do they reflect on the ability or integrity of those earlier workers whose theories have been superseded by more recent research using more refined techniques and starting with the advantage which even the existence of a wrong hypothesis gives to those who attack it. "All theories", writes Popper (*The Poverty of*

Historicism), "are trials; they are tentative hypotheses, tried out to see whether they will work . . . not only trial, but also error is necessary . . . all tests can be interpreted as attempts to weed out false theories."

In the fifteen years which have elapsed since Dr. Bowlby, in his brilliant paper on "Forty-four Juvenile Thieves" (1944), first drew attention to "maternal deprivation" as a strong factor in producing serious and persistent delinquents his theory has become one of the most widely discussed and accepted dogmas in the whole field of the social sciences, with correspondingly far-reaching practical consequences. Among those responsible for the care of children a tendency seems to have gained ground to regard early separation of a child from his mother as an evil to be avoided at any cost. It is only in recent years that a more discriminating attitude has emerged, and one of the most frequent criticisms has been concerned with the undue neglect of the role of the father which had been the almost inevitable, though perhaps not intended, consequence of the Bowlby theory. In the circumstances, it will be a matter of considerable interest to criminologists, psychologists, probation officers, child care and child guidance workers, and to institutional staffs everywhere to study Dr. Andry's book which I have the privilege to introduce to the public. Already in his work as a clinical psychologist in Australia, he had found the prevailing lack of interest in the part played by the father in the early training of children puzzling and dangerous, and he took the first opportunity which arose for him in this country to check the Bowlby hypothesis by way of careful systematic field studies. In the present book we are given the results of this painstaking investigation without any embellishments or exaggerated claims. Dr. Andry has been remarkably successful in obtaining first-hand information not only from the one hundred and sixty boys whom he personally interviewed, delinquents and non-delinquents (which latter term has now by general agreement been accepted as meaning "neither officially nor seriously delinquent"), but – at least for a smaller sub-group – also from their fathers and mothers. While the answers obtained from a lengthy Questionnaire were throughout exposed to the most rigorous statistical treatment, the statistical results are occasionally supplemented by clinical observations, and great care has been taken to check the consistency and meaningfulness of the replies. Proceeding patiently from one area of the whole field to another, the author has been able to build

up a revealing picture of parent-child relationships – a picture which
not only lends support to his own hypothesis that inadequacies of
the fathers were at least as responsible for the delinquent behaviour
of these boys as similar weaknesses on the part of their mothers, but
also illuminates certain far more general aspects of present-day
working class family life in a large city in this country. And as he
has not made the mistake of denying the mothers their due share it
might even be said that he has provided not only the anti-thesis to
the maternal deprivation theory but a synthesis as well.

HERMANN MANNHEIM
AUGUST, 1959

The London School of Economics
and Political Science
(University of London)

INTRODUCTION

This book, as its title implies, deals with certain aspects of family mental hygiene, and their relationship to delinquency. This involves the use of components from the two related fields of clinical psychology and criminology.

The central feature of the book is its concern with a problem that has much exercised the minds of workers in the field of delinquency namely, the playing of parental roles as one of the most important aetiological factors in the child's character formation.

It is generally nowadays accepted that well-played parental roles are a *sine qua non* to good mental health in children. In addition to this, however, much emphasis has in recent years been paid to the especially important role of the mother in this connection. The author, whilst not wishing to underestimate the importance of the maternal role, hopes to contribute to the study of delinquency in this book by drawing attention to the recently much-neglected study of *the role of fathers*.

The very great importance of the role of the father in relation to delinquent mal-adaptive behaviour, together with that of the mother, will become apparent in the following pages, which represent a preliminary study.

Part One

GENERAL INTRODUCTION

1 : THE BACKGROUND

A very large body of literature has grown on the subject of juvenile delinquency. In recent years the workers in this field have created some unanimity in concepts which enables them to use a common language and to use the accumulated knowledge as the starting-point for further elaborations of theory, research methods and therapy.

Viewing this vast volume of work, it would seem difficult, at first sight, for research workers to make essentially new contributions. However, the author, whilst claiming to make no revolutionary contribution to the study of juvenile delinquency, does feel that in the present work he has made a new contribution in that he shows the need for a change in emphasis in certain aspects of the theory of the aetiology of delinquency and shows the usefulness of a particular research technique, both as a pure research tool and as a clinical instrument.

But before going on to outline the aim of this study and the techniques used, the author would like to review three recent books which are of particular significance to his own study, and which in no small measure helped in the orientation of this study. This selection of of three books is in no way intended to minimize the value of other studies – some of the latter are briefly reviewed in Appendix 1.

Three Relatively Recent Key Studies

One of the more recent and best-known works in this field is that of Bowlby (1952) on *Maternal Care and Mental Health*. He points out that a child needs the warm feeling that derives from his relationship with his mother. If this is lacking, anxiety feelings are present and a state of 'maternal deprivation' develops. There may be partial or complete deprivation with resulting damage to the personality of the child. Partial deprivation causes acute anxiety and excessive need for love, and powerful feelings for revenge; whilst complete deprivation entirely cripples character development. Bowlby concludes that the following factors affect the extent to which damage may result in consequence of deprivation. (1) The age at which deprivation has occurred. (2) The length of deprivation. (3) The degree of deprivation.

3

(4) Frequency of deprivation. (5) Quality of mother-child relationships before separation. (6) The experience of a child with his mother substitute. (7) Kind of reception which the child receives from the mother on his or her return.

Bowlby lists some of the following disadvantageous after-effects following deprivation: (1) Hostility on the part of the child towards the mother on her return. (2) Excessive demands made on mothers followed by jealousy, temper tantrums, etc. (3) Cheerful but really shallow emotional attachment. (4) An apathetic withdrawal often accompanied by rocking and head-banging.

Deprivation is most damaging, Bowlby states, when a child is between the ages of 6–18 months. Periods less vulnerable in chronological order are the periods between 18 months to 3 years and 3 years to 5 years. Although still vulnerable, a child can survive deprivation from his 5th to 8th year with very little damage to character development.

Bowlby points out that three kinds of research techniques may be adopted to study deprivation: (1) Direct observation at the time separation occurs. (2) Retrospective studies, for instance, by carefully examining psychopaths and by delving into their early background. (3) Follow-up studies, i.e. longitudinal studies in which deprived children are observed growing up over a period of years.

It is, as yet, difficult to appraise fully Bowlby's most stimulating work, which in recent years has often been misquoted and misinterpreted. It should be remembered that further validation studies are still in progress under Bowlby's direction. A number of questions arise, however, which the writer feels need answering. One of the most important points is that the role of fathers has not been studied extensively by Bowlby, who has relegated the role of fathers to a secondary position to that of the mother, without having shown conclusively why this should be so. This omission is puzzling in view of the fact that Freud had much to say about the effect of fathers on the character development of children during the Oedipal stage. Furthermore, it is frustrating to find that some psychopaths and delinquents when examined do not appear to have had a history of maternal deprivation. It would seem difficult to assess accurately the many stages of deprivation, since individuals differ in their reactions to maternal separation as far as intensity, length and frequency of deprivation occur. Lastly, it should be pointed out that, by the very nature of his concepts, Bowlby's terms are difficult to define and to test objectively. There is, however, little doubt that Bowlby's work, more than most other previous works on parent-child relationships, has stimulated further research.

Another study which has had tremendous impact on researchers in the field of delinquency is that of Glueck and Glueck (1950) called *Unravelling Juvenile Delinquency* and more recently their *Toward a Typology of Juvenile Offenders* (1970). The Gluecks have contributed to the field of juvenile delinquency for approximately a quarter of a century. In this work they used a team of psychologists, psychiatrists, social investigators, anthropologists and statisticians. They matched non-delinquents with delinquents on a number of variables such as age, socio-economic background, I.Q., etc. They then investigated factors inside and outside the family structure of both groups and stress as one of the primary aetiological factors the major harm that may develop in a child if psychologically neglected by his parents. This 'under the roof culture' is thought to be more important than other factors, such as general environmental ones. The Gluecks have summarized much of the present knowledge about juvenile delinquency and have further confirmed a number of hitherto doubtful points regarding parent-child relationships. It should be noted, however, that their study may not be easily repeated. It must be borne in mind that the Gluecks have made great advances in this field through the publication of their prediction tables. These tables are based on their findings, and, according to the authors, are both reliable and valid and may be applied to any young offender who has not yet progressed far along the road of delinquency. The chance of any young offender's becoming a severe delinquent may be assessed by his score compared with that of the delinquents upon which the prediction tables were based.

The topic of prediction tables has recently come to exercise the minds of most workers in this field in the U.S.A., the United Kingdom and on the Continent (as evidenced by Fry's work, 1952).

Two works that must be mentioned are H. Mannheim's *Comparative Criminology* (1965), and Mannheim and Wilkins, *Prediction Methods in Relation to Borstal Training* (1955). The latter work is of specific interest from the point of view of methodology. Results of the validation study at once silence critics who query the possible value of the prediction tables. This work is largely based on the 'decision theory' which is an attempt to bypass concepts of causation and to re-emphasize the principle of practical operational research.

According to this theory, no causal hypotheses are necessary, and a research worker may use a set of data to derive a maximal system of control with respect to the end object via the possible decision. In bypassing aetiological concepts the authors do not deny the occasional use of such concepts, nor are they hostile to more familiar techniques which are employed in this field, such as the study of individual cases. The case-study approach and the prediction-table approach are not necessarily in opposition to each other, providing the case-study approach is objective.

Mannheim and Wilkins' (1955) approach to the study of juvenile delinquency is largely a utilitarian one in that the authors refrain from concentrating on aetiological questions but direct their research towards accurate predictions. Their study could be regarded as lying at one end of a continuum, whereas that of Bowlby's lies at the opposite end, since Bowlby's concentrates very largely on causative questions. The two approaches should be viewed as complementary to each other. Both works, together with that of the Gluecks, form a kind of triad since they approach the problem of juvenile delinquency in three different ways.

Current Studies

In bringing the original book of 1960 up to date, the author decided to stand back and add to the current edition some of the important works which have stood the test of time so far and which were mostly written either at the time the author carried out his research (presented here) or shortly afterwards. It is difficult to single out any particular work among many, the more so since doing this would merely reflect the slight shift of emphasis in the author's interest since he first began to work in this field over twenty years ago. However, in this connection, the following have particular relevance: (a) works relating to the field of group dynamic interaction between parents and children, or between others such as members working interdisciplinary teams in criminology, [R. G. Andry, *Forensic Psychology*, in preparation, and T. Grygier, J. C. Spencer, and H. Jones, *Criminology in Transition* (1965)]; (b) factor-analytical techniques relating to classification typology of offenders and the matching of personality of the treater and the treated (C. E. Sullivan, M. Q. Grant, and J. D. Grant, *Delinquency Integrations: 2nd technical report*, 1954), R. G. Andry's *The Short Term Prisoner* (1963); (c) the role partially played by constitutional factors, H. J. Eysenck, *Crime and Personality*

(1970), and G. Trasler, *The Explanation of Criminality* (1962); (d) techniques relating not only to psychoanalytical type of treatment especially related to the works of M. Klein (see A. Hyatt Williams in H. Klare and D. Haxby, 1967), but also to (e) behaviour therapy (H. R. Beech, *Changing Man's Behaviour*, 1969) and (f) chemotherapy (W. Sargant, *Battle for the Mind*, 1957; W. Sargant and P. Slater, 1964; John Pollitt, 1967), Eva Frommer, 1968, 1969. In addition might be mentioned certain texts which have set recent trends in criminology, psychology and sociology such as H. Mannheim's *Comparative Criminology* (1965), Howard Jones' *Crime and the Penal System* (1962), R. A. Cloward and L. E. Ohlin's *Delinquency and Opportunity* (1961), Donald West's *The Young Offender* (1967, 1969), Michael Argyle (1964, 1967, 1969), Nigel Walker's *Crime and Punishment in Britain* (1965, 1969), L. T. Wilkins' *Social Deviance* (1964), and J. E. Hall-Williams' *The English Penal System in Transition* (1970), Basil Bernstein's 'A Socio-Linguistic Approach to Social Learning' (1965), see also Denis Lawton (1969), M. E. Wolfgang and F. Ferracuti's *The Subculture of Violence* (1967), T. Sellin and M. E. Wolfgang's *The Measurement of Delinquency* (1964) and N. Morris and G. Hawker *The Honest Politician's Guide to Crime Control* (1969), P. Vernon's *Personality Assessment* (1964) and *Intelligence and Cultural Environment* (1969), and Roger Brown's *Social Psychology* (1965). A more detailed list of texts will be found in Appendix I which cannot itself be regarded as exhaustive in view of the ever increasing good texts appearing in this field.

2 : THE PRESENT STUDY

Many research workers, especially since the publication of Bowlby's previously mentioned work, have come to regard what is termed 'maternal deprivation' as being of primary aetiological importance in the fields of delinquency and psychopathology. The theory, in spite of its usefulness in special cases, can be criticized partly because it undermines the development of a theory based on interacting multi-causation and partly because it gives inadequate recognition (especially in view of Freud's findings) of the possible importance of the *role played by the father* – a role which complements that of the mother, forming a complex, subtle triangle of relationships between mother, father and child. The basic aim of the present work, then, is to study some important aspects of this triangle of relationships in certain key areas of the child's life experience – in other words, to study the role of *both* parents (and not merely that of the mother). It should be made clear here that the aim of the study is not to deny that the mother's role is important, but rather to investigate how important the father's role is *vis-à-vis* that of the mother's. Unless this is done, the primary importance or otherwise of the mother's role cannot be asserted. In short, the author does not believe that the theorists of 'maternal deprivation' have adduced sufficient evidence for their assumption of the essentially secondary role they attribute to the father.

The author felt that in order to carry out the task of examining the roles of both parents, considerable methodological rigour was required. The latter is often absent from clinical studies on the excuse that methodological rigour and subtle insight into complex human relationships are hard to combine. The author feels, however, that a truer statement of the position is that methodological rigour is often extremely hard to achieve in practice in any social research, and not that this necessarily conflicts with subtle insights. Thus, whilst he was fully aware of the difficulties, the author made every attempt to secure methodological rigour, in spite of many imperfections in the practical results of the attempt.

The research design was developed in the following manner.

First, the object of the research was defined. This was to investigate thoroughly the roles of *both* parents in order to determine whether differences exist between delinquents and non-delinquents in regard to the adequacy with which each parent plays his/her role.

Secondly, the decision was made to confine the research to a study of boys. The reasons for this decision were: (*a*) it is difficult to obtain girl delinquents for examination: (*b*) the majority of delinquents are boys: (*c*) since the study of the father's role was an important feature, of the research, and in view (according to Freudian theory) of the basic difference between boys and girls regarding emotional involvements with the father, girls were not studied in order to preclude over-complication of the findings.

Thirdly, in order to study subtle 'under the roof' relationships involved in the mother-father-child triangle, the decision was made to exclude boys from 'broken homes' from the research. Had the latter boys been included in the research, the pre-existing ill-balance in the family structure would have undermined the whole object of the research.

Fourthly, a series of interrelated hypotheses susceptible to empirical testing were set up regarding the adequacy of each parent's role in certain key areas of the life experience of the child. These hypotheses are set out in the relevant chapters of Part Two (The Findings) of this book and will not be further commented on here. A further set of hypotheses on the grandparents were set up, but it was found to be impossible to test them adequately; hence, no findings on these hypotheses are presented in this book. (The object of these latter hypotheses had been to establish whether there was any relationship between the roles of the boy's parents regarding him and the roles of the boy's grandparents regarding his parents when the latter were children, i.e. whether or not there was a transmission of parental attitudes from one generation to the other.)

Fifthly, a decision was taken as to what type of research should be used to test the hypotheses. It was determined that the research should be objective, quantitative and repeatable. These three criteria were essential if the hypotheses were to be properly tested and susceptible to independent testing by other research workers. Bowlby mentions three types of research which might be used in a study of this sort, namely, longitudinal or follow-up research, direct observation research, or retrospective studies. The ideal way, for instance, of studying 'maternal deprivation' and its consequences would be a combination of direct observation and longitudinal study. The research would start with direct observation of babies to see whether and how 'maternal deprivation' occurred, and then be followed by longitundinal studies over a period of years to see whether there was a greater tendency for 'deprived' babies to become delinquent than for 'non-deprived' babies. However, such ideal research is extremely difficult to operate and quite beyond the resources available to the author. He therefore had to resort to retrospective studies, as have most other research workers (including Bowlby, 1946) up till recently.

Having determined to use a retrospective study, the real work of research design itself started. In essence, the research design consisted of personal individual interviewing (by means of a formal interview questionnaire) of a test sample of 80 delinquent boys and a matched control sample of 80 non-delinquent boys. The reasons for and details of this design are given later in this chapter, but here two important points must be made.

i. Not only were the boys in each sample interviewed, but also *both* parents of a sub-group of 30 boys in each sample. The same questions (suitably re-phrased) were put to the boys and both parents with the aim of cross-checking the boys' responses. Many past studies have compared children's answers with those of their mothers, but it is believed that the present study is the first to compare concurrently the answers of fathers as well.

ii. Differences in parental roles between delinquents and non-delinquents were measured in terms of the *boys' perceptions* of the roles played by their parents and also in terms of the parents' perceptions of their own roles. The assumption behind the key concept of 'role perception' is that whether or not the *actual* roles of one or both parents highly correlate with the boy's *perceptions* of them, if the delinquent boys' perceptions of their parents' roles are highly negative and the non-delinquent boys' perceptions are positive, then a study of boys' perceptions of parental roles enables delinquents to be distinguished from non-delinquents.

Sample Design

As was previously indicated, a test sample of delinquents and a matched control sample of non-delinquents were selected. In spite of the difficulties involved in obtaining a matched control sample, it was felt that the latter was an essential feature of the research method, because otherwise there would be no indication of whether or not observed characteristics of the delinquents in the test sample were uniquely delinquent traits.

The sizes of the samples (and the sub-samples) were determined by the need for them to be sufficiently large for statistically significant results to emerge consistent with them being sufficiently small for one researcher to cope with (practical considerations connected with the structure and operation of the institutions in which the research was carried out also limited the sample sizes).

It was intended to select delinquents who were already fairly far advanced in criminality (in order clearly to distinguish the test sample from the control sample) and who were not mentally deficient or neurotic (inclusion of boys with the latter traits would have undermined the basis of the research – especially given the limited sample size). As regards advanced criminality, the type of institutions indicated were an Approved School or a Borstal. However, discussions with the Home Office showed that it would be extremely difficult to contact the parents of boys in such institutions; hence such institutions were not appropriate for this particular study. As a second choice various child guidance clinics were approached, but it was pointed out by the staffs that the number of suitable cases passing through the clinics was too small in the time available; further, many cases would display neurotic symptoms.

Discussions with the L.C.C. finally led to the selection of a Remand Home for boys in London. Thus the sample of delinquents, although not as advanced in criminality as boys in Borstals, were confirmed delinquents (in that they were referred to the Remand Home by juvenile court Magistrates for special psychiatric and psychological investigation, usually because they were recidivists). For the present study, the term 'delinquent' was operationally defined as: 'any boy who had more than one recorded Court offence to his name, who was referred for psychological investigation to the Remand Home because of his recidivision, and who was not considered to be neurotic, psychotic, or mentally defective'.

Further discussion with the L.C.C. led to the choice of two adjacent and similar secondary modern schools in a London borough as being the most appropriate institutions for securing a sample of non-delinquents. The borough was a working-class area with a high percentage of delinquency. The term 'non-delinquent' was operationally defined as: 'any normal boy who had never been brought before a juvenile court and had never attended a child guidance clinic, either because of stealing or because he was considered to be neurotic, or who because of persistent truanting had been brought to the notice of school authorities'. This definition deliberately does not exclude boys who might have stolen in the past or present but who have not been brought before a juvenile court – this was because it was felt that some stealing of a relatively harmless and non-persistent order is indulged in by many boys.

Group matching of the sample of delinquents and the sample of non-delinquents was carried out for a number of characteristics discussed below. A table showing the composition of the two samples is given after this discussion.

Geographical location: As has been pointed out, the two samples were in the London area. It was found that the delinquents in the Remand Home came from various working-class districts in London. Since there is no London area that can be considered to be purely delinquent or purely non-delinquent, although some areas have a higher delinquency rate than others, it was decided that non-delinquents should be selected from a working-class area with a high delinquency rate.

Age groups: Since the age ranges of boys at secondary modern schools (the location of the non-delinquent sample) and of boys at Remand Homes are from 11 to 15 years, the two samples were matched for each age between 11 and 15 years.

Intelligent quotient: It was decided that the boys in each sample should have an intelligence quotient between 80 and 125. It was felt that boys either side of this range would be atypical in their reactions to their parents' role playing and in their assessments and ability to communicate their assessments of their perceptions of parental role playing. The range also excluded mental defectives from the sample. Where the boys' I.Q.'s had not already been assessed by the schools or by the Remand Home, the author administered individual intelligence tests.

Mental state: The boys in each sample were non-neurotic and non-psychotic. It was easy to eliminate boys who were neurotic or psychotic from the delinquent sample by examining the psychiatrists' reports to Courts and the psychological assessments of the psychologist.

Socio-economic characteristics: The majority of boys in the Remand

Boys' characteristics in terms of social class and I.Q. within age

Ages	Total in each year	Hall-Jones social classes				Intelligence quotients			
		4	5	6	7	80–90	91–99	100–110	111–125
Delinquent total group									
12 years	28	1	13	7	7	14	7	7	–
13 years	11	–	4	2	5	3	4	4	–
14 years	13	1	7	4	1	2	5	5	1
15 years	28	1	9	9	9	9	7	10	2
All ages	80	3	33	22	22	28	23	26	3
Non-delinquent total group									
12 years	25	–	11	6	8	9	5	8	2
13 years	12	–	6	3	3	1	3	6	2
14 years	16	–	7	4	5	1	6	7	2
15 years	27	–	12	7	8	8	9	8	3
All ages	80	–	36	20	24	19	23	29	9
Delinquent sub-group									
12 years	8	–	5	1	2	6	1	1	–
13 years	5	–	2	–	3	2	1	2	–
14 years	6	–	3	3	–	–	3	3	–
15 years	11	–	2	5	4	4	–	6	1
All ages	30	–	12	9	9	13	5	12	1
Non-delinquent sub-group									
12 years	10	–	4	2	4	3	4	3	–
13 years	5	–	2	2	1	1	1	2	1
14 years	7	–	3	2	2	–	4	3	–
15 years	8	–	4	2	2	3	1	2	2
All ages	30	–	13	8	9	7	10	10	3

Home and in the two modern secondary schools were from working-class families. It was decided to eliminate all boys from middle-middle and upper-class homes from the two samples (using the Hall-Jones class categories). The two samples were matched for each of the Hall-Jones categories 4, 5, 6, and 7.

Family background: As was previously stated, all boys from broken homes were excluded from the two samples.

Questionnaire

Since the present study aimed at being objective, quantitative, and repeatable, it was felt necessary to conduct all interviews by means of a formal questionnaire – the latter being identical for all boys in each sample and being only (necessarily) slightly modified for parents (but the same for all parents).

Obviously this limited the depth to which the interviews could probe as compared with unstructured interviews, but the non-repeatability (and the much larger element of subjective influence by the interviewer) of the latter made it inappropriate for the present study. This was reinforced by the fact that the author hoped that interview questionnaire could be developed into a tool of diagnostic value to clinicians working in those child-guidance centres dealing mainly with juvenile delinquents and their parents. This latter desire and that for flexibility determined the use primarily of open-ended questions and also the ordering of the questionnaire.

The questions tended to be grouped to cover various fairly well defined areas relevant to the study. The aim was to present questions in an order least expected by the interviewee and also in an order that fluctuated in strength of effect (i.e., effectively changed groups of questions were interspersed by more neutral ones). The interview was begun by telling the interviewees that the interview was part of a study to find out differences in how people think in England as compared with say those in Australia – the object being to mask the real point of the study.

The interview questionnaire is given in full in Appendix 3 of this book.

Fieldwork

Delinquent boys, and the parents of the 30 boys in the sub-sample, were interviewed at the Remand Home. Non-delinquent boys were interviewed at their schools, and the parents of the 30 boys in the sub-sample were interviewed at their homes.

3 : THE FINDINGS

The objects of this chapter are:

i. to discuss the validity, reliability and interpretation of the findings obtained by the research technique used in this study;
ii. to outline the statistical method used in analysing the findings;
iii. to outline the procedure adopted in presenting the findings (in Part Two).

VALIDITY, RELIABILITY AND INTERPRETATION

It is necessary here to discuss three interrelated points on the general meaningfulness of the findings obtained by the particular research technique used in this study, namely:

i. How far are the findings a valid measure of what they purport to measure?
ii. How reliable are the findings?
iii. How far do the findings throw light on the causation of delinquency?

Validity

When constructing a questionnaire for use in research based on recall technique, it is difficult to find questions which will incontrovertably elicit 'the truth' *per se*. The aim becomes, then, to incorporate a 'self-validating' element into the questionnaire design, i.e. include questions which can be compared with some external criteria of truth. This can be done in two ways, namely:

i. by including 'factual questions' – questions whose answers can be checked against facts (e.g. 'What is your age?' or 'Where do you live?');
ii. by including questions whose validity has been shown by repeated past performances in other relevant studies.

The author eschewed both ways; the first because it is too *simpliste*, the second because, without denying the validity of other studies of

15

delinquency, the items used were not appropriate for testing the particular series of thematically interrelated hypotheses which the author felt he should test.

The author, in short, is attempting to break some new ground, hence the validity of his findings can only partly be assessed by comparison with past studies. Validation must await repeat performances of his study by other researchers.

Reliability

Valid findings *ipso facto* are reliable findings – findings cannot be valid unless they are reliable. Findings (and hence the research technique used to obtain them) are reliable if repeat performances of the study lead to substantially the same findings. If repeat performances are not possible (or, at least, not immediately) it becomes necessary to use some other method of testing the reliability of the findings (and, hence, the research technique). One well-known method of measuring the reliability of findings is to test their internal consistency. This might be done by comparing, for instance, the answers of one half of a given group with those of the other half of the same group. The author was able to do this in the present study by comparing the answers of all boys in each sample with those of the boys in the respective sub-samples (i.e. those boys whose parents were questioned). In the cases in which the author carried out such a comparison, a close similarity was found between the two sets of results. Hence, high reliability of the findings of this study can be assumed.

Interpretation

The present study was designed to highlight differences in the perception of parental roles between delinquents and non-delinquents. It was designed so that such differences would be highlighted by statistical analysis, but all the latter shows is whether observed differences could or could not have arisen by chance; it cannot state whether a causative factor is involved. Resolving this issue of causation is central to the whole interpretation of the findings.

Fortunately, the issue is resolved *as a first step* by decision theory (see Mannheim and Wilkins, 1955). According to this theory, consideration of causation does not have to arise in interpreting the results. If statistically significant differences are found to occur between two samples (e.g. delinquents and non-delinquents) and were obtained by an objective and repeatable research technique, then it must be assumed that such differences can predict behaviour and will continually differentiate between two groups. Causative studies can then follow. Determining what causal factors are involved in the differences in order to give meaning to the findings then becomes a further problem of interpretation – in much the same was as factors in factor analysis are interpreted in a meaningful way *after* the analysis has been completed.

Thus the author is primarily concerned with whether or not the adopted research technique can educe significant differences between delinquents and non-delinquents (mainly in relation to preception of parental roles) with a view to predicting future behaviour. However, the author is concerned with making a valid clinical study (which must have a statistically sound basis); hence the secondary qualitative interpretation of the quantitative findings is attempted.

METHOD OF STATISTICAL ANALYSIS
Significance Test

In order to determine whether or not the observed difference between the samples of delinquents and non-delinquents were significant or merely due to chance, recourse was had to the Chi-square (χ^2) test, The formula for Chi-square is:

$$\chi^2 = \sum \frac{(O - E)^2}{E}$$

that is, the sum of the squared differences between observed (O) frequencies and expected (E) frequencies divided by the expected (E) frequencies.

For reasons of expediency, the author analysed each observed difference to see whether it was above or below the 5% level of confidence and did not calculate separate levels of confidence for each observed difference. Hence, some of the findings given in Part Two of this book have a higher than 5% confidence level.

Calculation of χ^2

The answers of each group to each question were coded into a number of cells. To ensure no cell had a frequency of less than 5 (i.e. less than five boys in a given sample gave the coded answer) the most logically related cells were grouped together – an example is as follows:

Number of boys giving answer

	X	Y	Z	D	E	Q	M	B	C	GH
Delinquents	50	0	3	7	0	15	5	0	0	00	80
Non-delinquents	20	4	7	20	4	5	20	0	0	00	80

Having established the minimum cell frequency, the calculation was as follows:

i. number of degrees of freedom = number of groups – 1;

ii. the appropriate value of χ^2 at the 5% level for the degrees of freedom for each variable was obtained from a table of values of χ^2 (Table 5 in *Cambridge Elementary Statistical Tables*);

iii. the cell which, from inspection, appeared to make the greatest contribution to the ultimate value of χ^2 was then selected;

iv. the component was then calculated according to the formula:

$$\frac{(a - b)^2}{a + b}$$

where a is cell frequency in first row and b is cell frequency in second row;

v. if the value is 'iv' above exceeded that of 'ii' above, the distributions were significantly different at the 5% level;

vi. if the value in 'iv' did not exceed that in 'ii', the calculation was carried out (as in 'iv' above) for the group likely to give the next largest contribution to χ^2 – this value was added to the value in 'ii';

vii. if 'vi' was not greater than 'ii', then the above process was repeated until either a significant answer was obtained or the complete χ^2 had been calculated.

The procedure is admittedly not ideal, leading as it does to some not entirely happy groupings of cells (answers) in order to achieve statistical significance for inter-sample differences and leading to some differences not being given a high enough level of confidence. However, this useful procedure was adopted since the limited facilities and time of the author precluded more elaborate statistical tests.

PRESENTATION OF THE FINDINGS

The findings of this study are presented in Part Two of this book.

The findings consist of the results of tests on a series of interrelated hypotheses on differences between delinquents and non-delinquents chiefly regarding the playing of parental roles in key facets of the life experience of the boys. The attempt was made to group logically related hypotheses into eight chapters and to group logically related chapters into four sections. Because of the complex interplay of the factors studied, it cannot be claimed that the chapters and sections are discrete in themselves. A certain degree of arbitrariness with a pilot study of limited resources of this kind was necessary in allocating the hypotheses to chapters and the chapters to sections. However, it is felt that this necessary expository device, although involving some simplification of the issues involved, has not markedly distorted the findings and their implications.

Each section has an introduction outlining the areas to be discussed in its component chapters. Each chapter consists of three parts:

i. an introduction outlining the areas to be covered in the chapter;
ii. the findings of the tests of a series of hypotheses on facets of the area covered by the chapters;
iii. a summary of the findings.

Within each chapter's findings, each hypothesis covered consists of:

i. a statement of the hypotheses (on differences between the delinquent and non-delinquent group);
ii. A statement of the reasons behind the hypothesis;
iii. a statement of the questions by which the hypothesis was tested;
iv. a verbal statement of the quantitative results of the questioning and whether or not the hypothesis was confirmed;
v. a table showing the results of the questions in terms of number and percentages of the boys giving each answer and a statement of whether the apparent difference between the answers of the two groups of boys were statistically significant at the 5% level of confidence;
vi. a general commenting on the findings of the hypothesis.

In those chapters where the factors studied were sufficiently homogeneous, the findings concluded with the results of summary codes and parent-child agreement codes.

The sections and chapters of the findings are set out in the following order.

Section One is called 'The Emotional Atmosphere' and is concerned with the general emotional atmosphere in the home as perceived by the boys (and by their parents). This section consists of three chapters, namely:

i. Parental Affection – this is the key chapter of the study and presents findings on the parent-child affective relationships.
ii. Parent-Child Communication – which presents findings on 'environmental' and 'psychological' communication between parents and child (many of the factors studied in this chapter are intimately related to those in 'i' above and not easily separable from them).
iii. Home Climate – which covers certain factors not easily allocated to other chapters, but which seem best to include as part of the emotional atmosphere.

This section was placed first because the general emotional relationships covered were felt to be both a general condition and an active determinant of other aspects of the boys' general training in the process of socialization – as such the section was an essential prelude to the next section.

Section Two is called 'Training' and is concerned with aspects of parental training of the boys in infancy (primarily by the mother) and in later years (by both parents). The two stages of training are dealt with respectively in chapters entitled Infant Training and Later Training.

The first two sections of the findings were very much concerned with differences between delinquents and non-delinquents as regards their own (and their parents') perceptions of their parents' roles in the areas of life covered by these sections. The next section (Section Three) is called 'Consequences' and represents a shift away from the direct study of parental roles – it is concerned more with the consequences of the manner in which parental roles are played, namely, with certain aspects of the boys' behaviour. The two chapters in this section are:

i. Dynamics – which is concerned with differences between the two groups of boys as regards their reactions to stress situations and as regards the quantity and quality of their extra-familial social contacts – as determinants of a potentiality for delinquency.
ii. Delinquency – which is concerned with differences between the

two groups regarding specific deviant behaviour and parental reaction to such behaviour.

The last section (Section Four) is called 'Separation' and is concerned to take up issues of vital consequence to the theory of *maternal deprivation* – issues not covered in preceding chapters of the findings. It is also concerned with aspects of what could be called *paternal deprivation.*

Part Three of the book is made up of a chapter summarizing the study and another drawing conclusions from the study.

The Appendix (apart from the Questionnaire) forms a separate part of this study, and by concentrating on the review of the literature should help to provide the background against which this study has been set.

Part Two

THE FINDINGS

Section 1 : The Emotional Atmosphere

INTRODUCTION

As has already been stated, this study is concerned with:

i. parental roles in certain key areas of the life experience of the child;
ii. the child's perception of these roles.

This section is concerned with studying certain factors that make up the general emotional atmosphere in the home as perceived by the child. These factors are considered under three general headings, namely:

i. Parental Affection – which presents findings on which parent the child feels gives him the most affection (really the key factor in the whole of this study) together with related findings on, *inter alia*, the child's feelings as to the stability, degree and openness of parental love, which parent the child indentifies himself with, and the child's perception of parental hostility.
ii. Parental-Child Communication – which presents findings on what can be termed 'environmental' and 'psychological' communication between parents and child. 'Environmental' communication considers how far and in what way parents and child share leisure-time pursuits, and the child's attitudes to this. 'Psychological' communication considers which parent the child feels most understands him and which parent he turns to when in trouble.
iii. Home Climate – which presents findings on whether or not the child witnesses parental quarrels, and which parent is the more cheerful.

Again it must be emphasized that the multifarious factors considered in this study form a complex interacting whole and that, hence, some degree of arbitrariness is involved in disentangling them for separate study. Hence, no claim is made for the discreteness of the above headings. This section represents an attempt to study the previously mentioned subtle 'under the roof' relationships (and is not connected with the grosser forms of physical separation – i.e. 'broken homes'). Such relationships are a part, but also a general condition of the effectiveness of other parts, of the child's training in the general process of socialization. Thus this section, apart from its own intrinsic value, is an essential prelude to the next section (II) on parental training of the child.

1 : PARENTAL AFFECTION

This chapter is concerned with measuring the child's perception of his parents' affection for him with a view to establishing what differences, if any, occur between delinquents and non-delinquents. The factors studied here are obviously central to the author's intention to examine the affective roles of *both* parents and also represents an endeavour to test aspects of the validity of the theory that 'maternal deprivation' is of prime significance in the aetiology of delinquency.

1.1 *It is hypothesized that delinquents tend to feel loved more by their mothers than by their fathers, whereas non-delinquents tend to feel equally loved by both parents.*

The setting up of this hypothesis obviously derives from the author's view that the role of both parents needs reinvestigation, especially to observe the important role of fathers in the aetiology of delinquency. The hypothesis was directly tested by:

i. asking the simple question 'Which parent do you think loves you most – or you feel is a little closer to you?' (Q.8.12)
ii. asking, later, the question 'Who should love you more in the future?' (Q.8.16) – it being reasoned that if, for example, delinquents predominated in feeling more loved by their mothers than by their fathers, then they would predominantly answer that they should receive increased love from their fathers in the future;
iii. measuring the internal consistency (as an index of the reliability) of the answers to these two questions by comparing answers of boys in sub-group A with those of all boys (in both the delinquent group and the non-delinquent group.)

The internal consistency test was used here because the hypothesis is the central one of the area of parental affection – and, indeed, of the whole study.

The Results

The answers to the two questions are shown in the two parts of Table 1.1. The answers show that:

i. delinquents predominantly (69%) felt more loved by their mothers than by their fathers, whereas non-delinquents tended more to feel loved by both parents;

ii. half (54%) of delinquents felt that their fathers should love them more in the future, whereas the bulk (89%) of non-delinquents felt neither parent should love them more.

Thus the answers to the two questions are consistent with each other and both confirm the hypothesis (1.1).

Table 1.1: *Indications of which parent is considered to be more affectionate*

Which parent	Numbers		Percentages		
	Del.	Non-del.	Del.	Non-del.	
			%	%	
Loves boy most					
Mother	55	11	69	14	
Father	6	6	9	7	$\chi^2 > 7\cdot82$
Both[1]	12	45	15	56	significant
Others[2]	6	18	7	23	
Should love boy more					
Father	43	6	54	7	
Both	19	3	24	4	$\chi^2 > 5\cdot99$
Neither	18	71	22	89	Significant
Totals	80	80	100	100	

[1]includes 'both but mainly mother'
[2]includes 'don't know', 'neither', 'both but mainly father'

Table 1.SC (summary code of affection) following shows the results of the internal consistency test for the two test questions combined. The combination of the two questions was an attempt to devise an objective summary code of the whole area of parental affection based on two questions of high differentiating power between delinquents and non-delinquents – thus enabling the author to avoid making subjective evaluations of parent-child affective relationships.

The results show a high degree of agreement between the answers of sub-group A and the sample as a whole in the cases of both delinquents and non-delinquents. The differences between delinquents and non-delinquents within sub-group A and the total sample were of a similar order and statistically significant.

Table 1.SC: *Summary codes on adequacy of parental love for the total sample and for sub-group A*

Adequacy of parental love	Numbers		Percentages		
	Del.	Non-del.	Del.	Non-del.	
Total sample			%	%	
Both parents very satisfactory	9	62	11	78	
Mother or father satisfactory and other parent adequate	11	9	14	11	$\chi^2 > 5\cdot99$ significant
One or both parents very bad	60	9	75	11	
Total boys	80	80	100	100	
Sub-group A					
Both parents very satisfactory	5	25	16	84	$\chi^2 > 3\cdot84$ significant
One or other parent not satisfactory – usually father	25	5	84	16	
Sub-group A boys	30	30	100	100	

A Commentary

It is quite clear that the two simple questions had a high and internally consistent differentiating power as between delinquents and non-delinquents and that they confirm hypothesis 1.1. It would seem, therefore, that faulty *paternal* relationships rather than faulty *maternal* relationships primarily occur for the type of delinquent boy studied.

Aside from the statistical evidence given, it is worthwhile reporting some clinical observations of qualitative differences that emerged between delinquents and non-delinquents. It was found that there was a greater tendency for delinquents to 'block' emotionally on these questions on parental affection. Those who 'blocked' (in both groups) tended to say that they were loved by both parents. On the basis of pilot experience, it was decided that *all* boys who answered 'both parents' should be questioned once more (in a friendly but persistent manner). At this stage the two groups differed in their responses. Non-delinquents tended again to say they were loved equally by both parents (but thought mothers were of special importance to younger children). Delinquents, however, tended to show hostility and in many cases broke down and suddenly implicated one or other parent negatively (usually the father) – often with a notable display of affect.

1.2 *It is hypothesized that among both delinquents and non-delinquents, whichever parent is claimed to be the main protector now is also claimed to have been the main protector in the past.*

This hypothesis was set up in order to check the correctness and meaningfulness of hypothesis 1.1 (as to who is the most affectionate parent). As to the correctness of hypothesis 1.1, it was reasoned that there should be a high correlation between who is the most affectionate parent and who is the present main protector. As to the meaningfulness of hypothesis 1.1, it was reasoned that whatever the present family relationship may be it was not necessarily so, or recognized as such, in the past: hence, if hypothesis 1.1 were not to be misleading, it was necessary to demonstrate a continuity between perceived present and past behaviour. Hypothesis 1.2 was tested by asking all boys:

i. Which parent is more inclined to stick up for you even though you may be in the wrong? (Q.8.5)
ii. Has this always been so? (Q.8.6)

The acid test of this hypothesis was that the bulk of both delinquents and non-delinquents should affirm a continuity in the identification of their protectors.

The Results

Table 1.2 shows for both delinquents and non-delinquents:

   i. a high agreement between who is viewed as being the present protector (top part of table) and who is regarded as the most affectionate parent (see Table 1.1);

   ii. the overwhelming bulk of boys stating that the present protector has always been protective.

Thus hypothesis 1.2 is confirmed and, via the relationship between the most affectionate parent and the present protector, the correctness and meaningfulness of hypothesis 1.1 is confirmed.

Table 1.2: *Indications of continuity of parental affective roles*

Which parent is	Numbers		Percentages		
	Del.	Non-del.	Del.	Non-del.	
Present protector			%	%	$\chi^2 > 5 \cdot 99$ significant
Mother	63	31	79	39	
Father	8	13	10	16	
Both	9	36	11	45	
And in past					χ^2 not calculated. Not significant
Yes	74	79	93	99	
No	6	1	7	1	
Total boys	80	80	100	100	

A Commentary

It is apparent that both delinquents and non-delinquents perceive a continuity of parental behaviour as regards affective relationships, at least in so far as credence can be given to their statements as to the actual state of affairs. This finding is important in that most clinicians seem to agree that parental affection towards children requires stability and continuity in order to be most effective. However, the finding is primarily of importance to the central hypothesis of this study in that it tends to confirm the aetiological significance of faulty paternal affection in delinquency without the necessity of assuming an antecedent faulty maternal relationship. It is also important in giving cred-ence to the long-termness of the factors in other hypotheses pro-pounded in this study. In other words the questionnaire, in spite of its simplicity, appears to be elucidating long-term factors and not merely recent or transitory ones, and hence seems to be an effective test of the hypothesis.

1.3 It is hypothesized that the parents of delinquents show different degrees of affection from those of non-delinquents.

This hypothesis in part derives from hypothesis 1.1 (on who is the most affectionate parent) and hence its testing is a partial test of hypothesis 1.1. The hypothesis was also of interest in that it necessi-tated developing a technique of measuring degrees of affection. The Fels scales (Champney, 1941) were not considered appropriate to this particular problem and also had the disadvantage that the determi-nation of the degree of affection was left, to some extent, to the rater. The latter disadvantage was largely overcome in the present study by asking the following three questions (each question representing a rank order – or measurement – of degree of love):

i. Which parent may give too little love, affection and kindness to you? *(Q.8.14)*

ii. Which one of your parents is probably the one that gives the exact amount of affection to you? *(Q.8.15)*

iii. Which parent do you think loves you perhaps just a little too much than may be good for you? *(Q.8.13)*

The Results

Table 1.3 shows that:

i. only half (55%) of delinquents felt that neither parent gave too little love, whereas the bulk (96%) of non-delinquents felt this;

ii. only three-fifths (62%) of delinquents felt that the right amount of love was given by both parents, whereas the bulk (93%) of non-delinquents felt this;

iii. neither delinquents nor non-delinquents felt that either parent gave them too much love.

Thus hypothesis 1.3 is essentially confirmed.

A Commentary

The answers to *Q.*8.14 and *Q.*8.15 essentially confirm hypothesis 1.3 and are a further (partial) confirmation of hypothesis 1.1 (on who is the

Table 1.3: Indications of degrees of parental affection

Which parent gives:	Numbers		Percentages		
	Del.	Non-del.	Del.	Non-del.	
Too little love:			%	%	$\chi^2 > 3\cdot84$ significant
Mother or Father	36	3	45	4	
Neither parent	44	77	55	96	
Right amount of love:					
Father or both parents	30	74	62	93	$\chi^2 > 3\cdot84$ significant
Mother or neither parent	50	6	38	7	
Too much love:					χ^2 not calculated. Not significant
Neither parent	75	80	94	100	
Other answers	5	0	6	0	
Total boys	80	80	100	100	

most affectionate parent). The questions were also shown to be able to distinguish whether it was felt that too little love or the right amount of love was given by parents.

However, the answers to Q.8.13, whilst by no means negating the hypothesis, show the question to be inadequate for its task. This question was, in fact, difficult to score; it was found often to puzzle respondents. They tended to deny that parents ever habitually showed *too much* affection to a child, feeling excess affection to be more a sign of faulty discipline ('spoiling') rather than an inherent defect.

The results are also of interest in regard to the alleged ill effects of 'over protection of the child by the mother' (e.g. Levy, 1943; Newell, 1934, 1936) and demonstrate how difficult it is to devise an objective test to measure 'over-protection'.

The results tend to suggest that 'maternal over-protection' is not of primary importance in the bulk of delinquency inasmuch as 45 % of delinquents felt that both parents (hence, their mothers) gave them too little affection compared with only 4 % of non-delinquents who felt this.

1.4 *It is hypothesized that there is less mutual overt affection shown between parents and child among delinquents than among non-delinquents.*

It has often been posited in psychology that different kinds of affect-relationships between children and parents exist. For instance, there are some children who have very little feeling for their parents and give none overtly, some who have very little real feeling for their parents but can put on a show of affection (a 'hollow prince charming'), some who have warm feelings for their parents who are unable to give overt affection, some who have warm feelings and *are* able to give overt affection.

The testing of this hypothesis cannot directly show the existence of the types of children described above, since it relates only to overt display of affection (which may or may not be devoid of real content). However, it can throw light on whether or not:

 i. delinquents differ from non-delinquents in their ability to give overt affection;

 ii. parents of delinquents differ from parents of non-delinquents in the ability to give overt affection;

 iii. parents described as having difficulty in giving overt affection tend to have children who have the same difficulty.

The hypothesis is obviously of relevance to the concept of 'the affectionless character' as propounded by Bowlby (1946), but, owing to the already mentioned emphasis on overt affections, is not a complete test of that concept. Strictly speaking, the concept was not directly testable because it has not been clearly defined. The author felt that the concept could in part (and hypothesis 1.4 as a whole) be tested by the following questions:

 i. Is your mother the kind of person who gets rather embarrassed to show openly that she loves you? (Q.8.8)

 ii. Is your father the kind of person who gets rather embarrassed to show openly that he loves you? (Q.8.9)

 iii. Are you the kind of person who gets rather embarrassed to show openly that you love your parents? (Q.8.10)

The Results

Table 1.4 shows that:

 i. half (52%) of delinquents felt that their mothers were embarrassed to show open affection, whereas the bulk (88%) of non-delinquents did not feel this;

ii. two-thirds (65%) of delinquents felt that their fathers were embarrassed to show open affection, whereas three-quarters (77%) of non-delinquents did not feel this;

iii. nearly three-fifths (56%) of delinquents felt that they were embarrassed to show open affection to their parents, whereas the bulk (86%) of non-delinquents did not feel this.

Thus hypothesis 1.4 (on the lesser overt mutual affection among delinquents) is confirmed.

Table 1.4: Indications of openness of parent-child affection

	Numbers		Percentages		
	Del.	*Non-del.*	*Del.*	*Non-del.*	
Mother embarrassed			%	%	$\chi^2 > 3.84$
Yes	42	10	52	12	significant
No	38	70	48	88	
Father embarrassed					$\chi^2 > 3.84$
Yes	52	18	65	23	significant
No	28	62	35	77	
Boy embarrassed					$\chi^2 > 3.84$
Yes	45	11	56	14	significant
No	35	69	44	86	
Total boys	80	80	100	100	

A Commentary

Generally speaking, among both delinquents and non-delinquents the boys who had difficulty in showing affection openly to their parents also felt their parents had difficulty in showing affection openly to them (tending to implicate the father more than the mother). This implies a causative link between the parents' inability to express affection and that of the child.

Although the results are not inconsistent with Bowlby's (1946) findings and imply that delinquents tend to be more 'affectionless' than non-delinquents, it still remains that a substantial proportion of delinquents (44%) did not think they were embarrassed to show open affection (and both parents of most of this 44% agreed to this). Thus, although some positive relationship exists between inability to show affection and the evidence of delinquency, it seems safer to view each case on its merits rather than to affirm a general positive relationship.

1.5 *It is hypothesized that there is a greater tendency among delinquents to feel parental hostility towards themselves than among non-delinquents.* The tests of the hypotheses preceding the above one have shown that delinquents feel less loved by the parents (but mainly the father) than do non-delinquents. This naturally leads to the question of whether delinquents feel more parental hostility towards themselves than do non-delinquents. That is, does the deficient affective relationship imply merely a passive lack of parental love or positive parental hostility? Hypothesis 1.5 assumes the latter implication. The hypothesis was tested by asking the boys:

    i. If at all, which parent is inclined to nag a lot?   (Q.8.20)
    ii. If at all, which parent is inclined to pick on you?   (Q.8.21)

It was felt that these questions would also show the degree of parental hostility towards the child – 'nagging' being assumed to be a milder form of hostility than 'picking-on'.

The Results
Table 1.5 shows that:
    i. only two-fifths (42%) of delinquents felt neither parent nagged them, whereas the bulk (90%) of non-delinquents felt this;
    ii. two-thirds (63%) of delinquents felt neither parent picked on them, whereas the bulk (95%) of non-delinquents felt this.

Thus hypothesis 1.5 was confirmed.

A Commentary
Although the harsher form of parental hostility ('picking-on') was less widespread than the milder form ('nagging'), both forms of parental hostility were considerably more widespread among delinquents than non-delinquents. Thus, in the majority of delinquent cases, one or other parent is said to display positive hostility towards the boy.

Table 1.5: *Indications of degrees of parental hostility felt by the boys*

Which parent	Numbers		Percentages		
	Del.	*Non-del.*	*Del.*	*Non-del.*	
'Nags' boy most			%	%	
Mother	19	4	24	5	$\chi^2 > 5\cdot99$
Father or both	27	4	34	5	significant
Neither	34	72	42	90	
'Picks-on' boy most					$\chi^2 > 3\cdot84$
Either or both	30	4	37	5	significant
Neither	50	76	63	95	
Total boys	80	80	100	100	

1.6 *It is hypothesized that both delinquent and non-delinquents tend to feel that the more affectionate parents are the ones they most resemble in their looks and in their ways.*

This hypothesis was set up mainly in order to test a notion often advanced by clinicians that unconscious identification can be assessed by asking children which parent they think they look like and which parent they are like in their 'ways' (this latter expression is a colloquialism for an admixture of character and temperament). Such identification would shed light on one aspect of the formation of conscience and of character development in a child via identification (which may be positive or negative) with one or other or both of the parents. The ideal would appear to be a good identification of a boy with a masculine father. Delinquent behaviour might reflect a drastic falling away from this ideal.

The hypothesis was tested by cross-analysing the answers to Q.8.12 (which parent loves boy most) with each of the following questions:

i. Do you think that you look more like your mother (or her family) or like your father (and his family)? (*Q*.8.1)

ii. Whose ways do you have – your mother's or your father's?
(*Q*.8.3)

The Results

Table 1.6 shows:

  i. there was not an intimate relationship between the parent the boys felt most love them and the parent the boys felt they most resemble in looks (in that the 69% of delinquents who felt most loved by their mothers and the 86% of non-delinquents who felt most loved by the father or by both parents equally split 50/50 as to which parent they felt they most resemble in looks);

  ii. a much more intimate relationship was manifested between the most affectionate parent and the one felt to be resembled in ways (in that two-thirds of the 69% of delinquents who felt most loved

Table 1.6: Indications of boys' identification with parents

Parent who is most		Numbers		Percentages		
Affectionate	*Resembled*	*Del.*	*Non-del.*	*Del.*	*Non-del.*	
	in looks:			%	%	
Mother	Mother	28 ⎤	5	35 ⎤	6	
		⎱ 55		⎱ 69		$\chi^2 > 7{\cdot}32$
Mother	Father and Both	27 ⎦	6	34 ⎦	8	significant
Father and Both	Mother	9	34 ⎤	11	42 ⎤	
			⎱ 69		⎱ 86	
Father and Both	Father and Both	16	35 ⎦	20	44 ⎦	
	in ways:					
Mother	Mother	36 ⎤	4	45 ⎤	5	
		⎱ 55		⎱ 69		
Mother	Father and Both	19 ⎦	7	24 ⎦	9	$\chi^2 > 7{\cdot}32$
Father and Both	Mother	9	14 ⎤	11	17 ⎤	significant
			⎱ 69		⎱ 86	
Father and Both	Father and Both	16	55 ⎦	20	69 ⎦	
Total boys		80	80	100	100	

by their mother and four-fifths of the 86% of non-delinquents who felt most loved by their father or both parents said they resembled the more affectionate parent in their ways).

A Commentary

The results clearly do not support the hypothesis in respect of identification with the most affectionate parents via attributed resemblance in looks. However, the hypothesis is clearly confirmed in respect of identification with the most affectionate parents via attributed resemblance in 'ways'. It would seem then that this latter question (Q.8.3) can throw useful light on parental identification and on the total affective relationship between child and parents.

It is of interest to note that clinical observation showed several delinquents who stressed that they felt rejected by their fathers, pointing out negative characteristics which they reluctantly admitted to sharing with their fathers. Negative identification with fathers would seem to be the explanation here – one in keeping with the opinions expressed by Friedlander (1947) and Glover (1949) rather than with those expressed by the more extreme 'maternal deprivation' theorists (who appear to go beyond the defined position of Bowlby, 1952).

Parent-child Agreement Code

The summary code on affection (relating to Q.8.12 and 8.16) given in Table 1 SC was based on the boys' answers only. In the case of the sub-group A of each group, the summary code was applied to the answer of each parent of each boy. A comparison of the three summary codes (i.e. for the boy, mother and father) for each family gave the proportion of families showing complete agreement in answers to Q.8.12 and Q8.16 and showed whether the delinquent proportion differed from the non-delinquent proportion.

Table 1 AC shows that complete agreement occurred in the bulk of families in both sub-groups with no significant difference in the proportions in each sub-group.

Thus it would seem that deficient affective relationships between parents and boys are openly admitted on all sides in the delinquent group.

SUMMARY

In the first stage in an endeavour to determine what features in parental roles differentiate between delinquents and non-delinquents,

Table 1. AC: *Proportion of families in sub-groups showing agreement on who is the most affectionate parent*

Parent-child Agreement	Numbers		Percentages		
	Del.	Non-del.	Del.	Non-del.	
			%	%	$\chi^2 < 3{\cdot}84$
Complete	22	26	73	87	Not
Incomplete or none	8	4	27	13	significant
Total families	30	30	100	100	

certain aspects of the general affective relationships between each parent and the child were studied. The study of this area of the child's life experience is central to the whole of the study reported in this book, since good parent-child love relationships are a basic pre-condition and active determinant of the adequacy of parental role playing. Because the affective roles of both parents were studied, this chapter represents to some extent a fundamental test of the theory that 'maternal deprivation' is the primary factor in the aetiology of delinquency.

The findings of this chapter can be summarised as follows. Delinquents and non-delinquents were radically differentiated in their feelings as to the adequacy of the affective roles of the parents in that:

i. delinquents tended to feel that their mother loved them most, whereas non-delinquents tended to feel loved by both parents – thus the differentiating feature here was the inadequate love given by the father among delinquents;

ii. this last statement was reinforced in that delinquents tended to feel that their father should love them more, whereas non-delinquents felt that neither parent should love them more;

iii. on the above two basic points, there was substantial agreement between views of parents and boys;

iv. that the above differentiating features were not of recent origin was indicated by the fact that both groups implied that present parental roles were not basically different from those in the past (in that the present main protector of the child

was also the past main protector and the main protector
was highly related to the more affectionate parent);

v. delinquent boys tended to feel that their parents (but
especially their fathers) were embarrassed to show open
affection for them, whereas non-delinquents did not feel this;

vi. there was a tendency for delinquents, in contrast to non-
delinquents, to feel embarrassment at showing open love for
their parents – implying a causal link between parents' inability to show open love and that of the child;

vii. there was a tendency for delinquents to feel parental hostility
towards them (in terms of 'nagging'), whereas non-delinquents
did not feel this;

viii. there was a tendency for delinquents to feel that they had their
mother's ways rather than their father's ways, whereas non-
delinquents tended to feel they had both parents' ways or
their father's ways – thus indicating that delinquents tend less
to identify with their fathers than do non-delinquents.

Briefly these results can be summed up by saying that very strong evidence has been adduced for supposing that, in general:

i. delinquent boys receive less strong and open love from their
parents than do non-delinquents;

ii. it is the father's affective role that is (consistently) less satisfactory than the mother's among delinquents, in contrast to
the satisfactoriness of both parents among non-delinquents.

This last point throws considerable doubt on the theory that 'maternal
deprivation' is necessarily the primary determinant of delinquency, at
least, as far as delinquents who do not come from broken homes are
concerned. The theory of 'maternal deprivation' will be taken up in
detail in Section III (Separation).

Having established a case for believing that the inadequacy of father-
love at least as much as mother-love is what distinguishes delinquents
from non-delinquents, it is now necessary further to probe the 'emotional atmosphere' by examining whether or not differences occur
between the two groups as regards parent-child communication. In
view of the findings on affective relationships, it would seem reasonable to surmise that considerable differences between the two groups
would emerge, especially in regard to the role of fathers in the area of
parent-child communication.

2 : PARENT-CHILD COMMUNICATION

The concept of communication (i.e. between two or more persons) has long exercised the minds of psychologists, both in the academic field and in the child guidance field (e.g. Lewin, 1939; Moreno, 1956). It is a concept of considerable importance and value in describing relationships between persons, and constitutes here another important aspect, or area, of the family emotional atmosphere. The author found difficulty in delineating the area of communication because it interpenetrates with so many other areas (for example, it could be argued that parental-child affection is an aspect of communication). In practice, from *a priori* considerations, a number of activities and concomitant feelings were defined as belonging to the area of communication, and were then investigated. The author feels that it is often overlooked that two inter-acting aspects of communication can and should be distinguished, namely, environmental (or physical) communication and psychological (or emotional) communication.

It was felt that the adequacy of environmental communication could be measured by, for example, whether or not the child accompanied his father to football matches, or helped his mother at home, or spent much of his leisure time with his parents (e.g. in shared hobbies).

It was felt that the adequacy of psychological communication could be measured by whether or not the child felt understood by his parents and had confidence in his parents, and, hence, a desire to communicate with them by, for example, seeking their advice when in trouble.

In this area there are two basic hypotheses (referring, respectively, to environmental and psychological communication) and a number of derivative sub-hypotheses. It was the latter that were directly tested, each being a partial test of the relevant basic hypothesis. Hence, this chapter is divided into two parts; firstly, an outline of the environmental hypotheses and the test findings; secondly, an outline of the psychological hypotheses and the test findings.

Environmental Communication

The basic hypotheses here was as follows:

42

2.1 *It is hypothesized that parents of delinquents have less environmental communication with their children during leisure times than do parents of non-delinquents.*

Many students of delinquency have stressed the advantages which exist for children whose leisure-time activities are planned and the dangers which can accrue as a result of lack of parental supervision. It has been suggested that with failings on these counts children tend to join anti-social gangs, and that delinquency would decrease if parents spent more time with their children. The claim is that the 'good' parent, even if busy, *makes* time to spend with his child in order to communicate freely with him and set him a good example, thus helping him in the general process of socialization. It was therefore decided to set up test hypotheses on differences between delinquents and non-delinquents regarding:

  i. parental leisure time available for parent-child contacts;
 ii. whether or not the available leisure time was used for parent-child contacts;
iii. the quality of parent-child leisure-time contacts;
 iv. the boys' feelings about the adequacy of parent-child contacts.

These four sub-hypotheses to hypothesis 2.1 and the test results are set out separately in what follows.

2.1a *It is hypothesized that parents of delinquents tend to have less available leisure time than parents of non-delinquents because of work outside the home.*

One determinant of whether satisfactory leisure-time contacts occur is whether sufficient leisure time is available for such contacts. It is often alleged that poor communication exists between delinquents and their parents because the father's hours are more irregular and the mothers tend more to go out to work and to return later than those of non-delinquents. To test this sub-hypothesis the three following questions were put to the boys:

  i. Is your father very often on shift or overtime work, or on work that takes him away from home overnight? (*Q.2.6*)
 ii. Is your mother working at present – or has she done so up to the last few weeks? (*Q.2.1*)
iii. At what time does your mother come home after work? (*Q.2.4*)

Table 2.1a: Indications of whether or not outside work reduces the parents' leisure time for parent-child contacts

Answers	Numbers		Percentages		
	Del.	Non-del.	Del.	Non-del.	
Boys' answers: *Father on shift-work*			%	%	
Now or previously	24	12	30	15	$\chi^2 > 5.99$
Never	5	12	6	15	significant
Don't know	51	56	64	70	
Mother works					
Yes	38	41	48	51	$\chi^2 > 3.84$ not
No	42	39	52	49	significant
Mother returns home					
Before child	77	79	97	99	χ^2 not
After child	2	1	2	1	calculated.
Mother on night-work, leaves after supper	1	—	1	—	Not significant
Totals	80	80	100	100	
Parents' answers: *Father absent a lot for work reasons when boy was aged*					
6–15 (inclusive)	14	4	47	13	$\chi^2 > 3.84$
Don't know	16	26	53	87	significant
Total parents	30	30	100	100	

The Results

The answers in Table 2.1*a* show:

    i. limited knowledge on the part of boys on whether or not fathers did shift-work, but some indication from the boys – and strong indications from the parents that fathers of delinquents tend to do shift-work more than fathers of non-delinquents;

ii. approximately 50% of both groups had mothers who went out to work;

iii. only a negligible proportion of mothers are not at home before the children.

Thus hypothesis 2.1a was confirmed only in respect of fathers' shift-work being more widespread among delinquents.

A Commentary

Clearly the hypothesis is not substantiated as regards mothers, but is substantiated as regards fathers. Thus the oft-blamed factor for delinquency, that mothers are out working, is not here confirmed.

It is of interest to note that exhaustive questioning of a few cases, in both groups, of fathers who were supposedly on shift-work, etc., showed that shift-work, e.g., was sometimes an excuse for staying away from home, going to the pub.

2.1b *It is hypothesized that among delinquents less leisure-time parent-child contacts occur than among non-delinquents.*

The tests for hypothesis 2.1a indicated no strong evidence for assuming great disparity between delinquents and non-delinquents as regards the amount of leisure time which mothers possessed, but that fathers' leisure time was less among delinquents due to work duties. It is necessary, therefore, to enquire as to how far this available leisure time is used for parent-child contacts. The hypothesis was tested by asking the boys the following questions:

i. Do you prefer to be indoors at night? (Q.13.9)

ii. With whom do you spend most of your time when indoors? (Q.13.11)

iii. What do you usually do on Sundays? (Q.13.15)

iv. How much time do you and your mother spend together during week-ends compared with the time you spend by yourself? (Q.13.12)

v. How much time do you and your father spend together during week-ends compared with the time you spend by yourself? (Q.13.13)

The Results

Table 2.1*b* shows:

  i. that approximately three-quarters of both groups preferred to
     be outdoors at night;
 ii. only a tiny proportion (8%) of delinquents spent time mostly
     with parents when indoors, whereas 40% of non-delinquents
     said that they did so;
iii. only a fifth (20%) of delinquents spent their Sundays with their
     parents, whereas the bulk (86%) of non-delinquents said that
     they did so;
 iv. only a negligible proportion of delinquents spent more time
     with either parent than they did alone, whereas approximately
     seven-tenths of non-delinquents said that they did so;

Findings 'ii' to 'iv' essentially confirm sub-hypothesis 2.1*b* inasmuch
as delinquents do not appear to spend quite so much of their leisure
time with their parents.

A Commentary

Assuming that a preference for being outdoors generally will result
in boys spending much of their leisure time outdoors, then there was
an equal reduction in each group in the possibility of parent-child
contact. However, within this reduced possibility, parent-child contacts were far smaller among delinquents than among non-delinquents.

2.1c *It is hypothesized that the quality of parent-child contacts is lower
among delinquents than among non-delinquents.*

It has been shown that delinquents experience less parent-child (but,
especially, less father-child) contacts than do non-delinquents. It
remains to determine the quality of parent-child contacts. The hypothesis was tested by asking the boys the following questions:

  i. What kind of activities during leisure times do you and your
     mother share a lot?   (*Q*.13.5)
 ii. Do you and your father share many hobbies together?
                                                               (*Q*.13.6)
iii. What hobbies do you and your father share?   (*Q*.13.7)
 iv. Does your father often take you to outings such as football
     games, etc.?   (*Q*.13.1)

Table 2.1b: Indications of use of available leisure time for parent-child contacts

Answers	Numbers		Percentages		
	Del.	Non-del.	Del.	Non-del.	
Boy prefers to be indoors			%	%	
Yes	20	22	25	28	$\chi^2 > 3.84$
No	60	58	75	72	significant
How time is spent indoors					
Mostly alone	57	44	71	55	
Mostly with other children	17	4	21	5	$\chi^2 > 5.99$ significant
Mostly with one or both parents	6	32	8	40	
Sunday activity					
Visit or walk with parents	16	69	20	86	
Visit pictures alone	25	7	31	9	$\chi^2 > 5.99$ significant
Visit pictures with friends	39	4	49	5	
Time spent with mother					
More than alone	5	59	6	74	
Same as alone	22	17	28	21	$\chi^2 > 5.99$ significant
Less than alone	33	4	66	5	
Time spent with father					
More than alone	3	54	4	67	
Same as alone	18	16	22	20	$\chi^2 > 5.99$ significant
Less than alone	59	10	74	13	
Totals	80	80	100	100	

Table 2.1c: Indications of the quality of parent-child contacts in leisure time

Answers	Numbers		Percentages		
	Del.	Non-del.	Del.	Non-del.	
Activities with mother			%	%	
Helping in home	9	54	11	67	
Talking and playing	15	7	19	9	$\chi^2 > 5.99$
Seldom shares activities	56	19	70	24	significant
Whether hobbies shared with father					
Frequently or occasionally	13	62	16	78	$\chi^2 > 3.84$
Hardly ever	67	18	84	22	significant
Sorts of hobbies shared with father					
Indoor—e.g. stamp collecting	6	31	7	39	
Outdoor—e.g. fishing	6	24	8	30	$\chi^2 > 5.99$ significant
No hobbies shared	68	25	85	31	
Goes with father on outings					
Yes	15	63	19	79	$\chi^2 > 3.84$
No	65	17	81	21	significant
Totals	80	80	100	100	

The Results

Table 2.1*c* shows:

    i. only a small proportion (11%) of delinquents helped their mother in the home, whereas two-thirds (67%) of non-delinquents claimed to do so;

ii. only a sixth (16%) of delinquents shared hobbies with their fathers, whereas four-fifths (78%) of non-delinquents did so;

iii. a substantial proportion (30%) of non-delinquents shared active outdoor hobbies with their fathers;

iv. only a fifth (19%) of delinquents went on outings with their fathers, whereas four-fifths (79%) of non-delinquents did so.

Thus, hypothesis 2.1c is essentially confirmed in that the quality of parent-child contact was lower among delinquents than non-delinquents.

A Commentary

The quality of leisure-time contacts between father and boy was definitely lower among delinquents than non-delinquents. But as regards the quality of contacts between mother and boy, some caution is required. The author's impression was that many non-delinquents tended to give stereotyped replies when claiming to help their mothers in the home (often this was found not to be an honest reply), whereas delinquents were more honest in admitting that they did not help their mothers (presumably because they felt guilty after their recent misdemeanours).

2.1d *It is hypothesized that delinquents tend to feel deeply the need for more leisure-time contacts with their fathers, whereas non-delinquents tend to feel satisfied with their contacts with both parents.*

It was felt that the inadequacy of leisure-time contacts of mothers with their delinquents boy was less than that of the fathers and was to some degree compensated by their affective values being better than those of the fathers. It was therefore felt that boys would feel more in need of greater contacts with their fathers than with their mothers. Hypothesis 2.1d was tested by the following questions:

i. If he (the father) does not (take you to football games), why not? (Q.13.3)

ii. Should your father do this sort of thing, i.e. take you to football matches? (Q.13.2)

iii. Would it be helpful if your father saw a great deal more of you in the future? (Q.13.4)

iv. Would it be helpful if your mother saw a great deal more of you in the future? (Q.13.5)

Table 2.1d: *Indications of boys' feelings regarding
the adequacy of their leisure-time contacts with parents*

Answers	Numbers		Percentages		
	Del.	Non-del.	Del.	Non-del.	
Why not taken to sports by father			%	%	
Not applicable/ answered	25	63	31	79	
Boy considered too old now	7	7	9	9	$\chi^2 > 7.32$ significant
Father says he's too busy	36	5	45	6	
Father dislikes sports/doesn't care	12	5	15	6	
Should father take you to sports					
Yes	69	68	86	85	$\chi^2 > 3.84$ not significant
No	11	12	14	15	
Would it be helpful to see more of father					
Yes	65	10	81	13	$\chi^2 > 3.84$ significant
No	15	70	19	87	
Would it be helpful to see more of mother					
Yes	25	4	31	5	$\chi^2 > 3.84$ significant
No	55	76	69	95	
Totals	80	80	100	100	

The Results

Table 2.1*d* shows:

   i. three-fifths (60%) of delinquents attributed negative reasons on the part of their fathers for not taking them to sports;

ii. the bulk of both delinquents and non-delinquents felt their fathers should take them out to sports;

iii. four-fifths (81%) of delinquents, as against only an eighth (13%) of non-delinquents, felt it would be helpful to see more of their fathers.

iv. three-tenths (31%) of delinquents, as against a negligible proportion (5%) of non-delinquents, felt it would be helpful to see more of their mothers.

Thus sub-hypothesis 2.1*d* is confirmed in that delinquents tend deeply to feel the need for more contacts with their fathers.

A Commentary

The evidence strongly indicates that the fathers of delinquents gave reasons that were thinly disguised rationalizations for not taking their delinquent boys out. It is clear that delinquent boys, far from not caring about this lack of contact with their fathers, very much desired more contact with their fathers. Deep feelings on this were manifested by several delinquents who were near to crying and complained bitterly that their fathers never took them out, or, in some cases, took other siblings instead.

The desire by delinquents for more contact with their mothers, although more widespread than among non-delinquents, was by no means as great as their desire for more contact with their fathers.

Summary and Agreement Codes on Environmental Communication

It was felt that answers to questions 13.13 and 13.14 (on whether the boys spent more time alone or with each parent) most effectively showed the adequacy of parent-child environmental communication hence, a summary code and a parent-child agreement code was applied to these two questions.

Table 2.1 SAC shows:

i. that seven-tenths (71%) of delinquents indicated that both parents were unsatisfactory as regards environmental communication, whereas the bulk (85%) of non-delinquents felt both parents to be satisfactory;

ii. that the bulk of parents in both sub-groups agreed with their boys' evaluation of environmental communication.

Thus the delinquent boys tended to feel (and their parents tended to agree) that parent-child environmental communication was defective,

Table 2.1 SAC: *Summary and agreement codes on the adequacy of parent-child environmental communication*

Adequacy of environmental communication	Numbers		Percentages	
	Del.	*Non-del.*	*Del.*	*Non-del.*
Boys' estimates			%	%
Both parents very satisfactory	6	68	8	85
Mother satisfactory, Father just adequate/very unsatisfactory	17	7	21	9
Both parents very unsatisfactory	57	5	71	6
Totals boy	80	80	100	100
Parent-child agreement				
Complete	21	26	70	87
Incomplete or none	9	4	30	13
Total families	30	30	100	100

$\chi^2 > 5{\cdot}99$ significant

$\chi^2 < 3{\cdot}84$ not significant

whereas non-delinquent boys tended to feel (and their parents tended to agree) that parent-child environmental communication was satisfactory.

Psychological Communication

The basic hypothesis here was as follows:

2.2 *It is hypothesized that parents (but especially fathers) of delinquents have less psychological communication with their children during leisure time than do parents of non-delinquents.*

It was felt that a strong test of the general adequacy of psychological communication between parents and child would be whether or not the child would turn to its parents for advice when it was in trouble.

A sub-hypothesis on this was accordingly framed. However, in order to differentiate between the relative adequacy of fathers and mothers in each group in respect of psychological communication, further sub-hypotheses were set up on such factors as:

   i. which parent the boy feels most understood by;
  ii. which parent the boy turns to when he is in trouble;
 iii. which parent he prefers ultimately to deal with his case;
 iv. which parent he turns to first for general advice.

2.2a *It is hypothesized that delinquents, when in trouble, tend not to turn to their parents, whereas non-delinquents do so.*
Assuming the parents of delinquents were not themselves criminal, it was felt that one of the reasons why delinquents became delinquents was that when in trouble they felt that they could not turn to their parents for help and guidance. Hence, in trying to cope with their troubles by themselves, or in conjunction with inadequate guides (e.g. other boys), they further enmeshed themselves in trouble – eventually becoming classified as delinquents. The feeling that they could not turn to their parents when in trouble is an indication of defective parent-child psychological communication.

  This hypothesis was tested by the question:

    Are you inclined to consult your parents when in trouble, or do you try to wriggle out of it?   (*Q*.11.2)

The Results
Table 2.2*a* shows that the bulk (88%) of delinquents said that they did not turn to their parents when in trouble, whereas the bulk (86%) of non-delinquents said that they did so.

  Thus the sub-hypothesis 2.2*a* was confirmed.

A Commentary
The confirmation of this hypothesis clearly points to very inadequate parent-child psychological communications among delinquents.

2.2b *It is hypothesized that delinquents tend to feel more understood by their mothers than by their fathers, whereas non-delinquents tend to feel equally understood by both parents.*
It was felt that boys would tend to feel more understood by the more affectionate parent than by the less affectionate parent, hence the

Table 2.2a: Indications of whether or not boys turned to their parents when in trouble

In trouble, the boy	Numbers		Percentages	
	Del.	Non-del.	Del.	Non-del.
			%	%
Contacts parents	10	69	12	86
Tries to wriggle out of it	70	11	88	14
Total boys	80	80	100	100

$\chi^2 > 3\cdot84$ significant

wording of this hypothesis follows that of hypothesis 1.1 (on the most affectionate parent).

The hypothesis was tested by the question:

Which parent actually knows more about you?   (*Q*.11.1)

The question was deliberately vaguely phrased in order to cover, by implication, the boy's inner life as well as his overt words and deeds.

The Results

Table 2.2*b* shows that four-fifths of both groups felt more understood by their mothers than by their fathers.

Thus hypothesis 2.2*b* was not confirmed.

Table 2.2b: Indications of which parent understands the boy more

Boys more known by:	Numbers		Percentages	
	Del.	Non-del.	Del.	Non-del.
			%	%
Mother	65	62	81	78
Father	8	11	10	14
Both/neither	7	7	9	8
Total boys	80	80	100	100

$\chi^2 > 5\cdot99$ not significant

A Commentary

Two points should be made about the testing of this hypothesis. First, the author's probing of the boys' answers revealed that the majority had, as was hoped, interpreted the question to cover both their feelings and actions. Second, the boys felt that their mother understood them more because she saw more of them (at home) than the father, and therefore had a better opportunity to observe and study them. The few boys who felt their fathers understood them more than their mothers inferred that their fathers were more intelligent and often more capable than their mothers (e.g. 'Dad is very clever – he's always three jumps ahead of us – even though he's not always around', or 'Dad has all the brains at home, he always knows what we are up to').

2.2c *It is hypothesized that delinquents, when in trouble, tend to turn first to their mothers rather than to their fathers, whereas non-delinquents tend to turn to both parents.*

This hypothesis was set up like this because it was felt that when in trouble the boy would, if at all, turn first to that parent with whom he showed the best psychological communication (i.e. on the basis of hypothesis 1.1 and sub-hypothesis 2.2*b*).

This hypothesis was tested by the question:

> Which parent do you usually go to at first when you have done something wrong? (*Q*.11.3)

Table 2.2c: Indications of which parent is first turned to when boy is in trouble

Parent first turned to is:	Numbers		Percentages	
	Del.	Non-del.	Del.	Non-del.
			%	%
Mother	60	56	75	70
Father	9	11	11	14
Both	5	10	5	12
Neither	6	3	8	4
Total boys	80	80	100	100

$\chi^2 > 7.82$
not
significant

The Results

Table 2.2c shows tht the bulk of *both* groups turned to their mothers first when they were in trouble.

Thus hypothesis 2.2c was not confirmed.

A Commentary

A reason why both groups of boys tended to turn to their mothers first was that the mothers were the first available for consultation – this being reinforced in the case of delinquents by the fact that they had better emotional relationships with their mothers than with their fathers. Even with non-delinquents this would apply because though generally satisfied with the relationships with their fathers, they still felt closer to their mothers and used her as an intermediary with their fathers.

2.2d *It is hypothesized that delinquents, when in trouble, tend to prefer their mothers ultimately to deal with them, whereas non-delinquents tend to prefer their fathers to do so.*

It was felt that boys would tend to prefer ultimately to be dealt with by the recognised effective source of authority in the family providing they could expect reasonable fairness from this source – (a point that is further studied in Chapter 5). Previous hypotheses in this study (and those to be stated in Chapter 5) determined the phrasing of the above hypothesis.

This hypothesis was tested by asking the boys:

> Which parent do you prefer ultimately and finally to deal with your case if you have done something wrong?   (*Q*.11.)

The Results

Table 2.2d shows that three-fifths (60%) of delinquents preferred to be dealt with ultimately by their mothers, whereas three-fifths (57%) of non-delinquents preferred to be dealt with ultimately by their fathers.

Thus the hypothesis was confirmed.

A Commentary

In a sound family structure where the father is felt to be adequately affectionate and the ultimate source of authority (on the latter, see hypothesis 5.1 in Chapter 5), it would be expected that, although the

Table 2.2d: *Indications of which parent is preferred to deal ultimately with boy's wrong-doings*

Preferred parent	Numbers		Percentages	
	Del.	Non-del.	Del.	Non-del.
			%	%
Mother	48	19	60	24
Father	19	46	24	57
Both	9	9	11	11
Neither	4	6	5	8
Total boys	80	80	100	100

$\chi^2 > 7.82$
significant

mother may be first turned to by the boy when he is in trouble and used as an intermediary, the boy would prefer to be dealt with ultimately by the father. Where the father is not felt to be adequately affectionate and an effective authority, then it is not surprising that the boy still prefers his mother finally to deal with him.

2.2e *It is hypothesized that delinquents tend to go first to their mothers rather than their fathers for advice, whereas non-delinquents tend to go first to their fathers.*

The reasons for so phrasing this hypothesis are similar to those given for hypothesis 2.2d.

The hypothesis was tested by asking:

Which parent do you go to at first when you want some advice? (Q.11.7)

The Results

Table 2.2e shows that three-fifths (57%) of delinquents said they would go first to their mothers for advice, whereas half (46%) of non-delinquents said they would go first to their fathers. If the boys who said 'both parents' are taken into account, then only a quarter (27%) of delinquents as against three-quarters (76%) of non-delinquents would turn to their fathers for advice.

Thus the hypothesis was confirmed.

Table 2.1e: *Indications of which parents the boys turn to first for advice*

Boy first turns to:	Numbers		Percentages	
	Del.	Non-del.	Del.	Non-del.
			%	%
Mother	46	10	57	12
Father	14	37	18	46
Both	7	24	9	30
Neither	13	9	16	12
Total boys	80	80	100	100

$\chi^2 > 7.82$
significant

A Commentary

In view of the general trend of the findings so far in this study, the confirmation of this hypothesis is in no way surprising, in that the fathers of delinquents have been shown to play inadequate roles, especially as far as family leadership is concerned.

Summary and Agreement Codes on Psychological Communication

Summary and agreement codes were applied to questions 11.3, 11.5 and 11.7 – it being felt that answers to these most effectively displayed the degree of adequacy of parent-child psychological communication.

Table 2.2 SAC shows that as regards psychological communication:

i. only three-tenths (28%) of delinquents indicated that both parents were satisfactory of adequate, whereas two-thirds (64%) of non-delinquents indicated this;

ii. seven-tenths (72%) of delinquents indicated that their fathers were inadequate, whereas only a third (36%) of non-delinquents indicated this;

iii. few delinquents (less than 19%) and few non-delinquents (less than 30%) indicated that mother was inadequate;

iv. two-thirds of parents of delinquents and all parents of non-delinquents in the sub-groups agreed with their boys' evaluation of parent-child psychological communication.

Tables 2.2 SAC: *Summary and agreement codes on the adequacy of child-parent psychological communication*

Adequacy of psychological communication	Numbers		Percentages	
	Del.	Non-del.	Del.	Non-del.
Boy's estimates:			%	%
Both parents very satisfactory	11	41	13	51
Mother satisfactory but father just adequate	12	10	15	13
Mother satisfactory but father very unsatisfactory	42	5	53	6
Mother just adequate or both parents unsatisfactory	15	24	19	30
Total boys	80	80	100	100
Parent-child agreement:				
Complete	19	30	63	100
Incomplete or none	11	—	37	—
Total families	30	30	100	100

$\chi^2 > 7.82$ significant

χ^2 not calculable

Thus delinquents tended to feel (and their parents in the main agreed) that father-child psychological communication was inadequate, whereas non-delinquents tended to feel (and their parents agreed) that parent-child psychological communication was adequate.

SUMMARY

Following on a study of parental affective roles as perceived by the child (and largely confirmed by the parents), this chapter dealt with the interrelated factors termed parent-child communication. Two interacting aspects of communication were distinguished, namely, environmental and psychological and various facets of these were studied.

Environmental Communication

Summarizing the findings on environmental communication, it can be said that the distinguishing features between delinquents and non-delinquents in this area are:

i. fathers of delinquents tend to have less leisure time available (due allegedly to work duties) for contacts with their children than do fathers of non-delinquents (there were no significant differences between the groups as far as mothers were concerned);

ii. the quantity of leisure-time contacts between parents and child was much lower among delinquents than among non-delinquents;

iii. the quality of leisure-time contacts between parents and child was much lower among delinquents than among non-delinquents – this was definitely established as regards fathers of delinquents (less father-child sharing of hobbies and outings);

iv. that it was the fathers rather than the mothers of delinquents who were regarded as being most deficient in environmental communication, was indicated by the fact that the bulk of delinquents felt that it would be helpful if they could see more of their father, but the majority did not feel this about their mothers (the bulk of non-delinquents did not feel a need to see more of either parent).

In short, as the summary code showed, both parents of delinquents were viewed as inadequate by the boys in environmental communication, whereas both parents of non-delinquents were viewed as adequate (and the parents of each group tended to agree with these views). However, there were very strong indications that it was the father's defective roles that most troubled delinquents – which seems only natural since one would expect that a boy would desire positive leisure-time contacts more with his father than with his mother.

Psychological Communication

Summarizing the findings on psychological communication, the differentiating features were:

i. the bulk of delinquents tended not to contact their parents when in trouble, whereas the bulk of non-delinquents did so;

ii. delinquents tended to prefer their mothers to deal ultimately with their wrong-doings, whereas non-delinquents tended to prefer their fathers to do so;

iii. delinquents tended to turn to their mothers for general advice, whereas non-delinquents tended to turn to their fathers or both parents.

As regards which parent was felt to understand the boy most and which parent the boy turned to *initially* when in trouble, both groups gave a clear preference for their mothers – which means that these items do not differentiate between the two groups.

Briefly, then, as the summary code showed, the fathers' psychological communication was viewed as inadequate among delinquents, whereas both parents were viewed as adequate among non-delinquents.

Conclusions

Thus far, the findings have shown that, in relation to boys' perception of the roles played by their parents, the basic differentiating features between delinquents and non-delinquents are:

i. delinquent boys receive less strong and open love from their parents;

ii. delinquent boys experience less adequate environmental communication with their parents;

iii. delinquent boys experience less adequate psychological communication with their parents;

iv. on all the above three points, it is the father of delinquents who performs the most defective roles;

v. on all the above four points, the boys' parents substantially agree with the boys' views.

To complete the study of what has been termed 'the emotional atmosphere' (which is both a pre-condition of, and an active element in, the process of training the boys in socialization), the next chapter deals with some factors under the heading 'home climate'.

3 : HOME CLIMATE

This chapter is concerned with certain factors that are not easily allocated to other areas, but which can be subsumed under the (admittedly vague) term 'home climate' and, as such, forms part of this general section on the emotional atmosphere of the family. The home climate was measured by determining whether or not:

i. parents were generally cheerful;
ii. they quarrelled with each other in front of their children;
iii. the boys quarrelled with other siblings.

3.1 *It is hypothesized that among delinquents the mothers tend to be more cheerful than the fathers, whereas among non-delinquents the tendency is for both parents to be equally cheerful.*

It was felt that if both parents of a child were cheerful this would be conducive to a happier home atmosphere than if only one (or neither) parent were cheerful.

The hypothesis was tested by asking the boys:

Which parent is usually more cheerful at home?   (*Q*.9.3)

The Results

Table 3.1 below shows that seven-tenths (68%) of delinquents felt that their mothers were more cheerful than their fathers, whereas

Table 3.1: *Indications of which parent is more cheerful*

Which parent is more cheerful	Numbers		Percentages		
	Del.	*Non-del.*	*Del.*	*Non-del.*	
			%	%	
Mother	54	25	68	31	$\chi^2 > 3\cdot84$
Father	26	55	32	69	significant
Total boys	80	80	100	100	

seven-tenths (69%) of non-delinquents felt that both parents were equally cheerful or that their father was more cheerful. (Note: in both groups only a few boys said their father was more cheerful than their mother – these were combined with those saying 'both parents' in order to eliminate all frequencies of less than 5.)

Thus hypothesis 3.1 was confirmed.

A Commentary

Clearly, delinquents homes were less pervaded by parental cheerfulness than were non-delinquents homes, and the fathers of delinquents were clearly most to blame for this. In fact, there were indications that the more affectionate parent and the more cheerful parent tended to be one and the same person.

3.2 *It is hypothesized that there is a greater tendency among parents of delinquents than among parents of non-delinquents to quarrel with each other in front of their children.*

It has often been suggested that the home atmosphere of delinquents is considerably more tense than that of non-delinquents due to open arguments and even violent quarrels between parents of delinquents. This hypotheses was tested by asking the following questions:

   i. Do your parents often quarrel in front of you?   ($Q.9.1$)
   ii. Do your parents quarrel slightly more than average parents?
                                                 ($Q.9.2$)

The first question was deliberately so phrased as to assume that parents did quarrel.

The Results

Table 3.2 shows that the bulk of both delinquents and non-delinquents did not feel that their parents often quarrelled in front of them, or, indeed, quarrelled more than other parents.

Thus hypothesis 3.2 was not confirmed.

A Commentary

In spite of the deliberately phrased question, only a small proportion of either group appeared to come from homes where open dissension occurred. It seems probable that the open parental quarrelling which some writers have found associated with delinquency may apply to more advanced offenders (e.g. those in need of institutional care).

Table 3.2: Indications of degree of parental quarrels

Parents quarrel	Numbers		Percentages		
	Del.	*Non-del.*	*Del.*	*Non-del.*	
in front of boy			%	%	$\chi^2 < 3\cdot84$
Yes	12	6	15	8	not
No	68	74	85	92	significant
more than average					$\chi^2 < 3.84$
Yes	11	6	14	8	not
No	69	74	86	92	significant
Total boys	80	80	100	100	

Hence the association cannot, especially on the evidence of the present study, be generalized into applying to all delinquents: rather, as the previous two chapters have shown, a more subtle and pernicious influence than open and violent quarrelling appears to be at work.

3.3 *It is hypothesized that delinquents tend more than non-delinquents to quarrel with their siblings.*

This hypothesis does not refer to parent-child relationships; but the author's original intention had been to broaden its scope so as to throw light on which parents supported which child in inter-sibling quarrels.

Table 3.3: Indications of inter-sibling quarrels

Boy quarrels with	Numbers		Percentages		
	Del.	*Non-del.*	*Del.*	*Non-del.*	
			%	%	
No siblings	31	68	39	85	$\chi^2 > 3\cdot84$
One or more siblings	49	12	61	15	significant
Total boys	80	80	100	100	

The aim had been to elucidate, in addition to the amount of sibling quarrrels in each group, whether delinquents felt they were discriminated against by one or other parent, especially in relation to a sibling which the delinquent feared or disliked. However, the testing of such a wider hypothesis would have involved undue prelonging of the interviews. Hence, the above restricted hypothesis was postulated and then tested by asking:

> If at all, with which brother or sister do you seem to quarrel mostly? (Q.7.1)

The Results

Table 3.3 shows that three-fifths (61%) of delinquents quarrelled with one or more of their siblings, whereas the bulk (85%) of non-delinquents did not do so.

Thus hypothesis 3.3 was confirmed.

A Commentary

The hypothesis was confirmed, but it should be noted that no evidence of whether or not inter-sibling quarrels occur more in large families than in small families has been given. This limitation is important because delinquents do tend to come from larger families – a point which also links up with the author's original intention to give this hypothesis a wider scope. Some weak evidence on the relationship of inter-sibling quarrelling to large families is given by the fact that the 61% of delinquents who quarrelled were made up of 37% who came from large families (i.e. with five or more children) and 24% who came from smaller families.

Summary and Agreement Codes

Summary codes were not set up because of the heterogenous nature of the factors considered in this chapter. Inspection revealed (as was found to be the case in previous chapters) no substantial difference between the answers of parents and boys, hence, no agreement codes were devised.

SUMMARY

Superficially, the home climate, as measured by perceived parental quarrelling, would not appear to differ as between families of delinquents and families of non-delinquents. However, indications of greater home tensions among delinquents were manifested by two features:

   i. father of delinquents appeared to be less cheerful in the home (which would contribute to general tension);

  ii. inter-sibling quarrels were more rife in homes of delinquents.

Section Summary

Thus, summing up what has been termed 'the emotional atmosphere', the findings in this section have shown, that on the basis of the boys perceptions of their parents roles (and, indeed, on the basis of the parents' perceptions of their own roles), the following general points differentiate delinquents from non-delinquents:

   i. delinquents experience less open and strong love from their parents (especially from their fathers);

  ii. delinquents experience less adequate communication (both environmental and psychological) with their parents (especially with their fathers);

 iii. delinquents experience a more tense home atmosphere (to which their fathers contribute a substantial share);

In short, delinquents experience, in general, inadequate and tense emotional relationships with their fathers but very much less so with their mothers; whereas non-delinquents experience, in general, adequate emotional relationships with both parents.

  Thus far, then, the findings have not supported the theory that 'maternal deprivation' is necessarily the primary factor in the aetiology of delinquency (at least, in so far as the boys from broken homes are not implicated). They have also fully justified the author's claim that the role of *both* parents needed reinvestigation, and supported his view that the fathers' roles would seem to be of great aetiological significance in delinquency among boys.

  This chapter has completed the findings on the emotional atmosphere, hence it is now necessary to study parental roles in the process of the boys' socialization. This is done in the next section entitled 'Training'. It is worthwhile to emphasize once again that neither within or between chapters and sections are the factors under study to be considered as discrete and complete in themselves – they are merely artificial isolates constructed for the purposes of research and of exposition.

Section 2 : Training

The child's life experience determines how far he develops the kind of character which enables him to function relatively smoothly in the matrix of society around him. The various schools of psychology generally agree that effective socialization is dependent on a number of favourable conditions, such as:

i. adequate rapport between parents and child must exist so that the child feels sufficiently loved by his parents to make him feel the need for (to find meaning in) socialization – training and learning;

ii. a consistent mode of training based more on the positive approach of praise and reward rather than the negative one of punishment.

Condition 'i' above was studied in Section I where it was shown that in respect of delinquents the father's role was inadequate. It remains, therefore, to study the content and efficacy of the direct training in socialization to determine whether differences occur between delinquents and non-delinquents.

This is done under two general headings, namely:

i. Infant Training – which presents findings on the adequacy of breast-feeding and toilet training of the boys.

ii. Later Training – which presents findings on the source of authority in the family, and the system of reward and punishment in the family.

4 : INFANT TRAINING

It has long been stressed that inadequate parental care in the earliest stage of a child's life is likely to manifest ill effects in the child's later life. This chapter is concerned with studying whether or not material differences exist between delinquents and non-delinquents in respect of:

  i. adequacy with which they are breast-fed;
 ii. deviations from maturational norms in such factors as sitting up, walking, talking, and cutting of teeth.

The findings are based on the replies of mothers in the two special sub-groups (the replies of boys and fathers, as might be expected, being unreliable).

4.1 *It is hypothesized that mothers of delinquents were less adequate in breast-feeding their child than were mothers of non-delinquents.*

In testing this hypothesis, it was not possible to cover all the factors that go to make up adequate breast-feeding. However, three important factors were covered, i.e. whether or not the mother breast-fed the child, how long the child was breast-fed and whether or not the child was fed at regular intervals.

Current thought on the subject usually advocates breast-feeding up to nine months with feeding at regular intervals.

The hypothesis was tested by the following questions:

  i. Was your boy breast-fed?   (*Q*.6.1)
 ii. How old was your boy when breast-feeding stopped? (*Q*.6.2)
iii. Did you give your child milk whenever he cried or only at regular intervals?   (*Q*.6.3)

The Results

Table 4.1 following shows:

  i. approximately two-thirds of mothers of delinquents and of mothers of non-delinquents said they breast-fed their boy;
 ii. only a third (34%) of mothers of non-delinquents as against

68

three-fifths (60%) of mothers of non-delinquents said they breast-fed their boys for nine months or more;

iii. approximately four-fifths of both sets of mothers said they fed their boys at regular intervals.

Thus the hypothesis was confirmed only in respect of length of period of breast-feeding.

Table 4.1: Indications of adequacy of breast feeding

Answers	Numbers		Percentages		
	Del.	Non-del.	Del.	Non-del.	
Breast-fed or not:			%	%	$\chi^2 < 3.84$
Yes	19	21	63	70	not
No	11	9	37	30	significant
Period of breast-feeding					
Not applicable	11	9	37	30	$\chi^2 > 3.84$
Under 9 months	9	3	30	10	significant
Over 9 months	10	18	34	60	
When child fed					$\chi^2 < 3.84$
Whenever he cried	7	5	23	17	not
At regular intervals	23	25	77	83	significant
Total mothers	30	30	100	100	

A Commentary

The hypothesis was confirmed only very weakly in that mothers of delinquents tended to breast-feed their boys for a shorter period. Even this criterion of inadequacy is suspect because the alleged ideal of nine months is open to question and appears to be culturally and individually determined.

4.2 It is hypothesized that delinquents were more 'difficult' and retarded in infant maturation than were non-delinquents.

Workers in the child welfare and guidance field have often reported that a considerable proportion of mothers of delinquents have said their delinquent boys have been different from their siblings almost from birth. They would incessantly cry and be generally difficult and later become irritable and destructive. In view of this, the above hypothesis was set up and tested by such factors as to whether or not mothers felt their boys:

   i. had been 'cross' babies;

  ii. had been normal, retarded, or advanced in regard to bowel training, bladder training, sitting up, cutting of teeth, walking and talking.

The Results

Table 4.2 following shows:

   i. a small tendency for delinquents to have been 'cross' babies;

  ii. no difference between delinquents and non-delinquents as regards infant maturation. The bulk of mothers in both groups were claiming that their boys were normal on all counts.

Thus the hypothesis was not confirmed except on the weak count of a slight tendency for delinquents to have been cross babies.

It should be noted that no χ^2 was calculated on any result since inspection shows no differences between the two groups or the cell frequencies were less than 5.

A Commentary

Essentially, the hypothesis was not confirmed. However, it should be noted that mothers' answers to maturation questions tended to be stereotyped. This tendency was strengthened by the fact that the questions included the precoded answers 'normal', 'retarded' or 'advanced'. This limitation was unavoidable because more complex questions would have lengthened the already long questionnaire to an unmanageable degree (and would have shifted the centre of gravity of the research).

Summary and Agreement Codes

No summary codes were set up on Infant Training because the results show that the majority of hypotheses were not confirmed. No parent-child agreement codes were set up because, as would be expected, the answers of boys and fathers were not reliable.

Table 4.2: *Indications of infant maturation*

Answers	Numbers		Percentages	
	Del.	*Non-del.*	*Del.*	*Non-del.*
'*Cross*' *baby*			%	%
Yes	8	2	27	7
No	22	28	73	93
Bowel training				
Normal	29	30	97	100
Advanced	1	—	3	—
Bladder training				
Normal	29	30	97	100
Advanced	1	—	3	—
Sitting up				
Normal	28	30	93	100
Advanced	2	—	7	—
Cutting teeth				
Normal	27	30	90	100
Advanced	2	—	7	—
Retarded	1	—	3	—
Walking				
Normal	28	30	93	100
Advanced	2	—	7	—
Talking				
Normal	27	30	90	100
Advanced	1	—	3	—
Retarded	2	—	7	—
Totals	30	30	100	100

SUMMARY

The findings on infant training have shown only slight differences between delinquents and non-delinquents on two counts:

   i. delinquents tended to be breast-fed for shorter periods than non-delinquents;
   ii. a slightly larger proportion of delinquents than non-delinquents tended to have been 'cross' babies.

Thus, basically, no material differences in infant training was found between delinquents and non-delinquents.

5 : LATER TRAINING

As has already been mentioned the efficacy of training is conditioned by the emotional atmosphere in which it is carried out. Section I (The Emotional Atmosphere) has dealt with the basic factors of the latter, and it was shown that, generally speaking, the delinquent boy perceives his father as being markedly less adequate than his mother in this general area of life, whereas non-delinquents appeared to be generally content with both parents. Against this background, it is now necessary to enquire whether or not the child perceives a clear and stable source of authority in the family and a 'fair' system of rewards and punishments. It seems reasonable to suppose that if the child is confused as to the source of authority and as to the rationale of the rewards and punishments (due to parental emotional instability and inconsistency in disciplinary reactions to situations), then his character development will be such as to make his functioning in society less effective and more painful (for him and others). It is also felt that the better approach to training a child is the positive one of praise and reward of good behaviour rather than the negative one of punishment of bad behaviour. An overdose of the negative approach and an underdose of the positive approach would undermine the 'fairness' of training in the child's eyes.

This chapter sets up and tests hypotheses on differences between delinquents and non-delinquents on the following aspects of perceptions of parental training:

    i. whether or not a clear source of authority exists in the family;
   ii. the parents' reactions to trouble;
  iii. the 'reasonableness' of parents in regard to punishment;
   iv. the degree of strictness of parents;
    v. whether or not the parents give due praise to their boys.

5.1 *It is hypothesized that the fathers tend to be less clear sources of authority in the families of delinquents than in those of non-delinquents.*
It was hypothesized in Section I that the roles of the fathers of delinquents were inadequate in many emotional aspects of the life ex-

73

perience of delinquents. Given this, it seemed reasonable to suppose that this would reflect itself in the father's role as the prime source of authority in the family. Three constituents of authority were selected for study, namely, who the boy considers to be the ultimate head of his family, which parent is the main source of punishment, and which parent the boy tends most to obey.

As regards who is felt to be the ultimate head of the family, the author felt that the father would be considered to be the head of the family in London working-class homes – from which the samples in this study were drawn (this does not, of course, preclude the possibility that the situation differs in other areas of the country or in other cultures). It was felt that fathers of delinquents might be weak leaders and not the chief authority in their homes, or that they might assume leadership on some occasions but pass over leadership to mothers when they begin to lose interest in the structure and unity of the home.

It was felt that this would be reflected in which parent was the main source of punishment and in which parent is usually obeyed. In respect of these two aspects, it was felt that the father or both parents equally would tend to be implicated among non-delinquents, whereas the father's role would be defective among delinquents.

The hypothesis was tested by the following questions:

    i. Which parent has in fact the final say in your home? (Q.10.1)
   ii. Which parent mostly punishes you?   (Q.10.2)
  iii. Which parent do you usually obey at home?   (Q.10.10)

The Results

Table 5.1. shows:

    i. seven-tenths (71%) of delinquents and the bulk (85%) of non-delinquents felt their fathers or both parents had the final say in their homes – i.e. no significant differences between the two groups exist;
   ii. a greater proportion of non-delinquents than delinquents implicated both parents as the main source of punishment, but, although statistically significant, the difference is not of material significance in view of the small proportions involved in each group – combining the figures for fathers and both parents shows statistically no significant difference between the two groups;

iii. only a half (52%) of delinquents indicated father or both parents as being usually obeyed whereas the bulk (88%) of non-delinquents indicated this.

Thus the hypothesis that among delinquents' fathers tend to be less clearly the source of authority in the family than is the case with non-delinquents is essentially confirmed.

Table 5.1: Indications of source of authority in the family

Which parent	Numbers		Percentages		
	Del.	Non-del.	Del.	Non-del.	
			%	%	
Has final say:					
Mother	23	11	29	14	$\chi^2 < 5{\cdot}99$
Father	46 ⎫	57 ⎫	58 ⎫	71 ⎫	not
	⎬ 57	⎬ 69	⎬ 71	⎬ 86	significant
Both	11 ⎭	12 ⎭	13 ⎭	15 ⎭	
Usually punishes:					
Mother	19	19	36	24	
Father	45 ⎫	39 ⎫	56 ⎫	49 ⎫	$\chi^2 > 5{\cdot}99$
	⎬ 51	⎬ 61	⎬ 64	⎬ 76	significant
Both	6 ⎭	22 ⎭	8 ⎭	27 ⎭	
Is usually obeyed:					
Mother	28	6	35	7	
Father	28 ⎫	27 ⎫	35 ⎫	34 ⎫	$\chi^2 > 7{\cdot}82$
	⎬ 42	⎬ 70	⎬ 52	⎬ 88	significant
Both	14 ⎭	43 ⎭	17 ⎭	54 ⎭	
Neither	10	4	13	5	
Total boys	80	80	100	100	

A Commentary

Whereas non-delinquents very strongly tend to recognise their fathers as the head of their families and to obey them most, delinquents strongly tend to recognize their fathers as head of their families but to obey them least. Thus, as perusal of Table 5.1 shows, the effective head of the family (measured in terms of boys' obedience) is as likely to be the mothers as it is likely to be the fathers. This points to a greater degree of defective paternal leadership among delinquents than non-delinquents.

These findings are fully consistent with those found in the sub-hypothesis on psychological communication in Chapter 2.

5.2 It is hypothesized that there is a greater tendency among delinquents to feel their parents show over-emotional reactions to trouble than among non-delinquents.

It was felt that parents of delinquents would tend to give vent to more emotional displays than show calm reason over troubles than would those of non-delinquents, this being functionally related to inadequacies in the general parent-child emotional relationships and the inadequate definition of authority in the family.

The hypothesis was tested by the following questions:

    i. Which parent is rather too quick-tempered and flares up when he or she hears of trouble? (*Q*.10.15)

    ii. Which parent usually keeps cool and reasonable during trouble? (*Q*.10.16)

    iii. Which parent keeps it up too long after the trouble has been dealt with (doesn't forgive)? (*Q*.10.17)

    iv. Which parent does not keep it up long enough after the trouble has been dealt with (forgives too quickly)? (*Q*.10.18)

The Results

Table 5.2 shows:

    i. the bulk of boys in both groups implicated one or other of their parents as being too quick tempered in their reactions to trouble – but there were no significant differences between the groups as to which of their parents were implicated;

    ii. over half (54%) of delinquents felt their mothers kept cooler than their fathers, whereas non-delinquents split more or less equally on which parent kept cooler;

    iii. under half (46%) of delinquents felt neither parent 'kept it up too long', whereas nearly two-thirds (63%) of non-delinquents felt this – further, delinquents tended more to implicate their fathers as keeping it up too long;

    iv. the bulk of boys in both groups did not feel that their parents did not 'keep it up' long enough.

The hypothesis that parents of delinquents show greater emotional reactions to trouble than those of non-delinquents was only weakly confirmed by points 'ii' and 'iii' above.

Table 5.2: Indications of parental emotional reactions to trouble

Which parent:	Numbers		Percentages		
	Del.	Non-del.	Del.	Non-del.	
Is too quick-tempered:			%	%	
Mother	21	29	26	36	$\chi^2 < 7.82$
Father	46	33	58	41	not
Both	6	5	7	6	significant
Neither	7	13	9	7	
Keeps cool:					
Mother	43	31	54	39	
Father	16	28	20	35	$\chi^2 > 7.82$
Both	8	15	10	19	significant
Neither	13	6	16	7	
Keeps it up too long:					
Mother	13	17	16	21	
Father	30	13	38	16	$\chi^2 > 5.99$
Neither	37	50	46	63	significant
Does not keep it up long enough:					
Mother and/or Father	15	12	12	15	$\chi^2 < 3.84$ not
Neither	65	68	88	85	significant
Total boys	80	80	100	100	

A Commentary

The hypothesis can hardly be said to have been confirmed. However, if it were modified to refer to fathers of delinquents as being more over-emotional, then it would be more strongly confirmed in that a smaller proportion of fathers of delinquents appear to keep cool and a greater proportion appear to 'keep it up too long' than of fathers of non-delinquents. However, even then the hypothesis would not be strongly confirmed.

5.3 *It is hypothesized that parents of delinquents tend to show less 'reasonableness' in regard to punishments than do those of non-delinquents.*

Parental 'reasonableness' in regard to punishments of the boys was felt to be functionally related to the adequacy of general parent-child emotional relationships, to the parents' emotional reactions to trouble, and to the authority structure in the family. The hypothesized deficiencies in families of delinquents as regards the factors naturally led to the above hypothesis. The hypothesis was tested by the following questions:

i. Which parent often threatens with punishment but never quite carries it out in the end?   (*Q*.10.7)
ii. Which parent usually carries out punishment after a previous warning has been given?   (*Q*.10.8)
iii. What kind of punishment works best with you?   (*Q*.10.12)

The Results

Table 5.3 shows:

i. no significant differences between the two groups as regards non-executed threats of punishment;
ii. only a third (32%) of delinquents said that their fathers carried out punishments after a previous warning, whereas three-fifths (59%) of non-delinquents said this;
iii. only a negligible proportion (5%) of delinquents said that just a talking to by their parents was the most effective punishment, whereas two-fifths (38%) of non-delinquents said this.

Thus, the hypothesis was (but not strongly) confirmed in that (*a*) fathers of non-delinquents tended more than those of delinquents to give a warning before punishment and (*b*) less negative punishments (i.e. being hit and being kept in) were effective with non-delinquents.

A Commentary

In so far as differences emerged as to which sort of punishment was felt to be most effective by the boys, there were indications of the

Table 5.3: Indications of parental 'reasonableness' in punishments

	Numbers		Percentages	
	Del.	Non-del.	Del.	Non-del.
Which parent makes empty threats:			%	%
Mother	41	44	51	55
Father	15	16	19	20
Both	19	7	24	9
Neither	5	13	6	16
Which parent gives previous warning:				
Mother	23	16	29	20
Father	26	47	32	59
Both or Neither	31	17	39	21
Which punishment works best:				
Being hit	39	26	49	32
Being kept in	21	16	26	20
Being talked to	4	30	5	38
Others	16	8	20	10
Total boys	80	80	100	100

Annotations at right of table:
- Which parent makes empty threats: $\chi^2 < 7{\cdot}82$ not significant
- Which parent gives previous warning: $\chi^2 > 5{\cdot}99$ significant
- Which punishment works best: $\chi^2 > 7{\cdot}82$ significant

history of parental 'reasonableness' in punishments. Thus, generally speaking, good training of a boy should mean that he does not require (or feel that he requires) strong punishments (e.g. being hit or being kept in) in order to behave reasonably satisfactorily. The fact that a larger proportion of delinquents than non-delinquents feels that the stronger punishment is more effective (more necessary) with them indicates that parents of delinquents have been less successful in establishing an effective 'reasonableness' than parents of non-delinquents in regard to punishment.

5.4 *It is hypothesized that there is a greater tendency among delinquents than among non-delinquents for one or both of their parents to be either too strict or too lenient.*

The functional relationships mentioned in the previous hypotheses in this chapter were felt to hold here, and gave rise to the wording of this hypothesis. The testing of the hypothesis naturally required a means of measuring the degrees of strictness involved. Again, the use of rating scales was foresworn in favour of the following questions:

  i. Which parent is rather too strict at home?   (Q.10.4)
 ii. Which parent is just right regarding strictness at home?
                                                          (Q.10.6)
iii. Which parent is rather too lenient at home?   (Q.10.5)
 iv. Which parent should be stricter in your home in future?
                                                          (Q.10.9)

The first three questions above form a ranking order of degrees of strictness. The last question above provides a check on the third question above.

The Results

Table 5.4 shows:

  i. due to exigencies of cell groupings the findings on which parent the boys felt was too strict were (although shown as statistically significant) of no material value;
 ii. two-thirds (66%) of delinquents felt that *neither* parent was just right as regards strictness, whereas four-fifths (81%) of non-delinquents felt that *both* parents were just right;
iii. only a fifth (21%) of delinquents felt that neither parent was too lenient, whereas three-fifths (61%) of non-delinquents felt this (delinquents tended more to imply that their mothers were too lenient rather than their fathers);
 iv. only a fifth (21%) of delinquents felt that neither parent should be stricter, whereas the bulk (87%) of non-delinquents felt this (delinquents strongly tended to feel that their mothers should be stricter rather than their fathers).

Thus, the hypothesis that parents of delinquents, in contrast to those of non-delinquents, tend not to strike the right balance as regards strictness was essentially confirmed.

A Commentary

Clearly, in the boys' eyes, parents of delinquents, in contrast to those of non-delinquents, tend not to achieve the right degree of strictness

Table 5.4: Indications of degrees of parental strictness

Which parent	Numbers		Percentages		
	Del.	Non-del.	Del.	Non-del.	
Is too strict:			%	%	
Father	21	5	26	6	$\chi^2 > 3\cdot84$
Mother or neither	59	75	74	94	significant
Is just right in strictness:					
Mother	10	5	13	6	
Father	8	5	10	6	$\chi^2 > 7\cdot82$
Both	9	65	11	81	significant
Neither	53	5	66	7	
Is too lenient:					
Mother	24	17	30	21	
Father	12	8	15	10	$\chi^2 > 7\cdot82$
Both	27	6	34	8	significant
Neither	17	49	21	61	
Should be stricter:					
Mother or both:	47	4	59	5	$\chi^2 > 7\cdot82$
Father	16	6	20	8	significant
Neither	17	70	21	87	
Total boys	80	80	100	100	

in handling their boys. Delinquents tend to imply that their mothers in particular are too lenient and, to a lesser extent, that their fathers are too strict. This, one suspects, links up with the findings of the section on The Emotional Atmosphere, where it was seen that the emotional father-child relationship was particularly defective among the delinquents. Where such relationships are poor it seems reasonable to assume that a delinquent would not like to see it aggravated further by an over-punishing father.

It is of interest to note that during the interviews the author found that most non-delinquents smiled when they admitted their mothers were too lenient, whereas delinquents made such admissions with a serious face as if aware that their mothers' leniency had been harmful to them. No such differences in behaviour between the two groups was noted in respect of fathers' strictness.

5.5 *It is hypothesized that delinquents tend to feel insufficiently praised by their fathers, whereas non-delinquents tend to feel sufficiently praised by both parents.*

An essential feature of training a child in socialization in that it should be based on a positive approach of praise and reward rather than on a negative approach of punishment. Which approach is used would be highly conditioned by the affective relationship between parent and child. It was, therefore, felt that the tendency to defective father-child affective relationships among delinquents would be manifested in a tendency for fathers to give insufficient praise to their boys.

This hypothesis was tested by cross analysing the answers to $Q.18.12$ (on the most affectionate parent) with those to the following questions:

i. Which parent praises you more often when you have done something well? ($Q.10.13$)
ii. Which parent should in future praise you more often if you have done something well? ($Q.10.14$)

The Results

Due to the exigencies of all groupings the data in Table 5.5 do not fully provide a quantification of the hypothesis.

The bottom half of the table does clearly bring out that only a third (32%) of delinquents as against the bulk (87%) of non-delinquents felt that neither parent should praise them more often in the future. This confirms the second half of the hypothesis. As regards which parent of delinquents was defective in praise it can be taken that a high correlation existed between the most affectionate parent and the one giving most praise. The wording of the table (because of necessary cell groupings) does not bring this out, but perusal of the raw data does. Because of this correlation, it follows that fathers of delinquents were defective in their praise of their boys. This confirms the first half of the hypothesis.

Table 5.5: Indications of which parent praises boy most

Which parent		Numbers		Percentages		
		Del.	Non-del.	Del.	Non-del.	
Loves most:	*Praises most:*			%	%	
Mother and/ or Father	Mother or Father	45	24	56	30	
Mother and/ or Father	Both or Neither	18	11	22	14	$\chi^2 > 7.82$ significant
Both	Mother or Father	11	29	14	36	
Both	Both or Neither	6	16	8	20	
Loves most:	*Should praise more*					
Mother and/ or Father	Father or Mother	46	7	58	9	
Mother and/ or Father	Neither	17	28	21	35	$\chi^2 > 7.82$ significant
Both	Father or Mother	8	3	10	4	
Both	Neither	9	42	11	52	
Total boys		80	80	100	100	

A Commentary

Thus once again it is the fathers' defective roles (in this case, in respect of praise) that serves to differentiate delinquents from non-delinquents – which is not surprising in view of this study's findings on other functionally related aspects of parental roles.

Summary and Agreement Codes

Summary and agreement codes were applied to questions 10.6 and 10.13 since it was felt that answers to these questions best typified the findings of this chapter.

Table 5.SAC shows that, as regards later training of the boys by parents:

   i. only one-tenth (10%) of delinquents indicated both parents as being satisfactory and seven-tenths (69%) indicated both parents

as being unsatisfactory, whereas the bulk (87%) of non-delinquents indicated both parents as being satisfactory;

ii. in both sub-groups, the parents, in the main, agreed with their
boys' evaluation (with no significant differences between
groups).

*Table 5.SAC: Summary and agreement codes
on the adequacy of later parental training of boys*

Satisfactoriness of training	Numbers		Percentages		
	Del.	Non-del.	Del.	Non-del.	
Boys' estimates			%	%	
Both parents very satisfactory	8	70	10	87	
One parent satisfactory, the other just adequate or unsatisfactory	17	6	21	8	$\chi^2 > 5.99$ significant
Both parents unsatisfactory	55	4	69	5	
Total boys	80	80	100	100	
Parent-child agreement					
Complete	21	26	70	87	$\chi^2 < 3.84$ not significant
Incomplete or none	9	4	30	13	
Total families	30	30	100	100	

Thus, delinquents tended to feel (and their parents, in the main,
agreed) that their parents' later training of them was inadequate,
whereas non-delinquents tended to feel (and their parents, in the
main, agreed) that their parents' later training of them was adequate.

SUMMARY

As a prelude to the study of the parents' training of their boys,
Section I studied three broad components of the emotional atmosphere of parent-child relationships, namely, general parent-child

affective relationships, parent-child communication (both environmental and psychological) and the home atmosphere. The findings showed that delinquents experience, in general, inadequate and tense emotional relationships with their fathers but very much less so with their mothers; whereas non-delinquents experience, in general, adequate emotional relationships with both parents.

In the light of these findings and of the general agreement among psychologists that effective training in socialization is conditioned by the adequacy of parent-child emotional relationships, the findings of the present chapter are not surprising. In brief, it was found that the chief differentiating features between delinquents and non-delinquents were:

i. among delinquents there was a tendency for their fathers not to appear clearly as the effective leader of the family, whereas among non-delinquents their fathers clearly appeared as effective leaders of the family;

ii. among delinquents there was a greater tendency for fathers rather than mothers to display over-emotional reactions to trouble than was the case with non-delinquents;

iii. among non-delinquents there was a slightly greater tendency for parents to show reasonableness in meting out punishments than among delinquents (fathers of delinquents being more implicated here);

iv. among delinquents there was a very marked tendency for parents not to strike the right balance as regards strictness (mothers in particular tending towards leniency) whereas among non-delinquents the bulk of parents did strike the right balance;

v. delinquents strongly tended to feel that they should receive more praise from both parents (but especially the father), whereas non-delinquents strongly tended to feel that they received enough praise.

In short, as the summary and agreement code showed, the parental roles in training their boys were markedly inadequate among delinquents (the fathers being particularly implicated) and generally satisfactory among non-delinquents.

Section Summary

The findings so far in this study of parental roles in certain key areas of the life experience of boys have shown that (on the basis of the boys' perceptions of their parents' roles and on the parents' perceptions of their own roles) delinquents are differentiated from non-delinquents in the following broad respects:

i. delinquents experience less open and strong love from their parents (especially from their fathers);
ii. delinquents experience less adequate communication (both-environmental and psychological) with their parents (especially with their fathers);
iii. delinquents experience more tense home atmosphere (to which their fathers contribute a substantial share);
iv. delinquents experience less adequate training (via punishments and rewards) from their parents (especially from their fathers).

Hence, thus far in the study of parental roles, it has been shown that parents of delinquents are less adequate than those of non-delinquents in certain key areas of the boys' life experience – but that it is fathers of delinquents who are especially inadequate. These findings, without denying that the mothers' roles are important, have served to highlight the great importance of the fathers' roles in the aetiology of delinquency – a point usually ignored in past studies of delinquency.

Thus far, the findings have concentrated on the differentiating features of delinquents and non-delinquents as regards parental role (as perceived by the boys and by their parents). In the next section, its two component chapters will study the consequences of these differences in terms, respectively, of certain aspects of social behaviour and of specifically delinquent behaviour.

Section 3 : Consequences

So far, this study has been concerned with determining what differences exist between delinquents and non-delinquents in those areas of their life experience that can be termed as family relationships (primarily, in terms of parental roles as perceived by the boys and by their parents). If a child experiences inadequacies on its parents' (but especially its father's) part in respect of love, communication (especially during emotional crises, and training, then, as a result of these faulty family relationships, the possibility is heightened for the child to develop a behaviour pattern that makes him prone to delinquent acts (e.g. aggressive reactions to difficult situations, less and poorer quality extra-familial social relationships) and, ultimately, to develop into a delinquent.

These possible consequences of faulty family relationships are studied under two general headings, namely:

i. Dynamics – which studies some features of the boys' possible behaviour which, although not delinquent as such, might determine whether or not they are predisposed to delinquency.

ii. Delinquency – which studies some features of the boys' possible behaviour which is more specifically delinquent and their parents awareness of and reactions to this behaviour.

Thus, this section departs from previous ones in that it is not primarily concerned with a study of parental roles but with possible consequences of ineffectively played parental roles.

6 : DYNAMICS

The findings so far have shown that delinquents suffer from more defective general emotional relationships with their parents and less adequate general training from their parents than do non-delinquents. It seems reasonable to infer that, apart from their specifically delinquent behaviour, such differences in the life experiences of delinquents and non-delinquents would tend to lead to differences in their behaviour. This chapter is concerned with studying some of these differences. Two aspects of behaviour were studied which were felt to be ultimately related to a potentiality for delinquent behaviour, namely, reactions to stress situations and general sociability.

6.1 *It is hypothesized that delinquents tend to have more aggressive reactions to stress situations than do non-delinquents.*

By an admitted simplification, it can be said that an individual who has been blocked or thwarted by a 'barrier' in achieving his goal has essentially only a limited number of possibilities open to him, (cf. Lewin *et al.* 1934), namely:

i. to show signs of aggression in an attempt to gain his goal by force;
ii. to show signs of 'regression' (in the Freudian sense) by becoming withdrawn or introspective in an attempt to compensate privately for the threatened loss of the desired goal (a neurotic ego defence machanism);
iii. to use 'detour behaviour', i.e., to forgo a frontal assault and adopt instead an outflanking move with aim of eventually gaining the original goal.

It was felt that, because they do not feel emotionally secure (due to defective parental love and general poor parental-child communication) and because of inadequate training and guidance from parents, delinquents are less able to cope with stress situations in a rational and/or socially minded manner than are non-delinquents. It was felt, therefore, that delinquents would tend to adopt an aggressive course of behaviour when faced with a situation they did not like, whereas non-delinquents would tend to have recourse to 'detour behaviour'. Since gross neurotics had virtually been eliminated from both samples (at the selection stage) it was not felt that delinquents studied would adopt markedly noticeable regressive behaviour.

It was also felt that aggressive behaviour if thwarted would be more likely to lead to the nursing of grievances and, hence, that delinquents would tend less than non-delinquents to get over distress caused by a disliked situation. It was felt that a big stress situation is punishment by parents and that aggressive behaviour would be manifested in resentment of this. If the parental system of rewards and punishments is felt to be 'fair' by the boy and operates in a context of a sound parent-child emotional atmosphere, it seems reasonable to assume that the boy will not greatly resent parental punishment. Since delinquents feel less loved (especially by the fathers, who usually administer the punishments), it was reasoned that delinquents tend to resent parental punishment.

There aspects of the hypothesis were tested by the following questions:

   i. When you seem to come up against something you do not like, how do you react? (Q.12.1)
   ii. How soon do you get over it – quickly or not? (Q.12.2)
   iii. How much do you seem to resent punishment from your parents? (Q.12.4)

The Results

Table 6.1 shows:

   i. only three-tenths (30%) of delinquents did not feel angry when they came up against something they did not like, whereas the bulk (88%) of non-delinquents did not feel angry (note that only 14% of delinquents tended towards regressive behaviour, i.e. got sulky or withdrawn);
   ii. most of both groups got over the disliked situation quickly;
   iii. two-thirds (65%) of delinquents openly or secretly resent parental punishment, whereas the bulk (84%) of non-delinquents did not do so.

Thus, on the more basic points 'i' and 'iii' above, the hypothesis that delinquents tend to be more aggressive in stress situations is essentially confirmed.

Table 6.1: Indications of reactions to stress situations

	Numbers		Percentages		
	Del.	Non-del.	Del.	Non-del.	
When boy dislikes situation:			%	%	
Gets rather angry	45	5	56	6	
Gets very sulky	11	5	14	6	$\chi^2 > 5\cdot99$
Does not feel very angry	24	70	30	88	significant
Gets over disliked situation:					
Quickly	56	63	70	79	$\chi^2 < 3\cdot84$ not
Not quickly	24	17	30	21	significant
When punished by parents:					
Resents it openly or secretly	52	13	65	16	$\chi^2 > 3\cdot84$
Not resentful	28	67	35	84	significant
Total boys	80	80	100	100	

A Commentary

Clearly delinquents were more inclined to aggressive behaviour than non-delinquents. Whereas the latter generally adopted 'detour behaviour', delinquents tended to be aggressive – but only to a small extent to be regressive. This finding is in substantial agreement with other writers who have stressed the aggressive element in the behaviour of delinquents. It was also confirmed by parents of delinquents who often complained that their boys seemed very resentful when punished (whereas parents of non-delinquents did not say this).

6.2. *It is hypothesized that delinquents tend more than non-delinquents to feel that they resemble their fathers rather than their mothers in their reactions to stress situations.*

It has often been postulated by previous writers that many delinquents come from homes where the parents are short-tempered and are resentful and aggressive when thwarted and that delinquents have probably copied such behaviour from their parents. Assuming that fathers of delinquents are more aggressive and less affectionate than those of non-delinquents, the above hypothesis naturally followed.

The hypothesis was tested by the question:

Which parent are you more like in this way? (i.e. in reactions to disliked situations). (Q.12.3)

The Results

Table 6.2 shows that approximately half of each group felt they resembled their father in their reactions to stress situations. Further, delinquents divided almost equally in attributing resemblance either to their fathers or their mothers. These results mean that hypothesis 6.1 was not confirmed.

Table 6.2: Indications of resemblance between parent and child to stress situations

Boy's reactions resembles those of:	Numbers		Percentages		
	Del.	Non-del.	Del.	Non-del.	
			%	%	
Mother	34	28	43	35	$\chi^2 < 5.99$
Father	38	42	47	52	not
Both	8	10	10	13	significant
Total boys	80	80	100	100	

A Commentary

Clearly delinquents did not feel themselves to be particularly like their fathers from the point of view of aggressiveness. In this connection one is driven to consider the many different types of delinquents and delinquency producing homes which must undoubtedly exist but in this complexity have been deliberately excluded from this study. For instance, the trouble of some delinquents may be that their fathers are too aggressive, whereas with other delinquents it may be that their fathers were too non-aggressive and had damagingly weak personal strictness.

6.3 *It is hypothesized that the tendency is for delinquents to have less numerous, and lower quality, extra-familial social contacts than non-delinquents.*

If, as has been hypothesized in earlier chapters, delinquents feel less loved and receive less adequate general parental training than non-delinquents, it seems reasonable to infer that they will tend to have less self-confidence and less self-discipline and that this will manifest itself in delinquents having less rich (in number and quality) social contacts outside their family than non-delinquents.

This hypothesis was tested by the following questions:

   i. Do you prefer to play with other children or to keep to your-
     self?   (*Q*.12.5)
  ii. What do you do when you are out-of-doors?   (*Q*.12.6)
 iii. Do you attend Sunday School, or Church, or Church Club?
                                           (*Q*.12.7)

The criteria selected for testing the hypothesis were not exhaustive, but time prevented more questions on more exhaustive criteria.

The Results

Table 6.3 shows:

   i. only a small proportion of either group preferred to play by
     themselves rather than with other children;
  ii. seven-tenths (72%) of delinquents said they roamed the streets
     with their mates, whereas over a half (55%) of non-delinquents
     said they went to a club or played cricket;
 iii. only a small proportion of either group attended Sunday School,
     etc.

Thus, hypothesis 6.3, on the greater poverty of outside social contacts among delinquents than among non-delinquents, was not confirmed in respect of there being more social isolates among delinquents, but was partly confirmed in the quality of such contacts.

A Commentary

Although the hypothesis was not confirmed in terms of significantly more social isolates occurring among delinquents than non-delin-

Table 6.3: Indications of extra-familial sociability

	Numbers		Percentages		
	Del.	Non-del.	Del.	Non-del.	
Boys prefer to:			%	%	
Play with others	63	71	79	89	$\chi^2 > 3\cdot84$
Play alone	17	9	21	11	significant
Boys out-of-doors activities					
Goes to pictures or club	6	27	8	34	
On street alone (on foot or bike)	8	7	10	9	$\chi^2 > 7\cdot82$
Roams streets with mates	58	29	72	36	significant
Plays cricket	8	17	10	21	
Boy attends Sunday School, Church, etc.					
Yes	12	15	15	19	$\chi^2 > 3\cdot84$
No	68	65	85	81	significant
Total boys	80	80	100	100	

quents, there was some evidence that the latter tended to use their time more constructively than delinquents. However, it is not to be inferred that the fact that the majority of delinquents roamed the streets with their mates means that they necessarily indulged constantly in illegal activities in gangs when out-of-doors. After all, a substantial proportion of non-delinquents also roamed the streets with their mates and the delinquents freely and cheerfully admitted their street-roaming activities.

Summary and Agreement Codes
Summary codes were not set up because of the heterogenous nature of the factors considered in this chapter. Inspection indicated no

major discrepancies in either group between answers of parents and boys, hence no agreement codes were set up.

SUMMARY

Summarizing the findings presented in this chapter it can be said:

i. delinquents tend more than non-delinquents to be aggressive in their reactions to stress situations as shown by their own admitted tendencies to feel anger when they come up against something they do not like;

ii. in line with 'i' above, delinquents also tend more than non-delinquents to resent parental punishment;

iii. delinquents tend no more than non-delinquents to copy their fathers' reactions to stress situations;

iv. whilst delinquents did not appear to be much more prone to social isolation than non-delinquents, it does appear that their outside social activities are probably not as constructive as those of non-delinquents.

7 : DELINQUENCY

The previous chapter dealt with one aspect of the consequences of parental role playing, namely, the boys behaviour in stress situations. This chapter also deals with the consequences of parental role playing, but with certain aspects of behaviour more directly associated with delinquency, The factors studied, on which hypotheses were framed and tested, were differences between delinquents and non-delinquents in respect of:

    i. the proportion of boys who indulged in truanting;
    ii. the proportion of boys who indulged in stealing;
    iii. the onset ages of truanting and of stealing;
    iv. parents' awareness of and reactions to their boys' deviant behaviour.

7.1 *It is hypothesized that a much greater proportion of delinquents than of non-delinquents have resorted to acts of truanting and of stealing at some time or other, and started to do so at an earlier age.*

The Gluecks (1950), and most other researchers have found a close correlation between the onset of truanting and stealing and have found that the earlier the onset of deviant behaviour, if it persists, the less favourable is likely to be the prognosis.

The hypothesis was tested by the following questions:

    i . How old were you when you first traunted?   (*Q*.4.1)
    ii. How old were you when you first started to take things that did not belong to you?   (*Q*.4.3)

These questions were deliberately so phrased as to assume that everyone had truanted or stolen at some time or other – the author's tone of voice when asking this question was also in keeping with this assumption.

The Results

Table 7.1 shows:

    i. the bulk (88%) of delinquents said that they had truanted at some time, whereas only half (46%) of non-delinquents had done so;

ii. the bulk (95%) of delinquents said that they had stolen at some time, whereas only two-thirds (68%) of non-delinquents had done so;

iii. as the data is presented in the table, it appears that delinquents tended to have started truanting and stealing at an earlier age than non-delinquents (another view of this data is given in 'a commentary' below).

Thus the hypothesis that truanting and stealing are more widespread and starts at an earlier age among delinquents than among non-delinquents is confirmed.

Table 7.1: *Indications of extent and onset age of deviant behaviour*

When boys first:	Numbers		Percentages		
	Del.	Non-del.	Del.	Non-del.	
Truanted:			%	%	
6–8 years	21	14	26	17	
9–11 years	30	7	38	9	$\chi^2 > 7.82$
12–14 years	19	16	24	20	significant
Never	10	44	12	54	
Stole:					
6–8 years	21	16	26	20	
9–11 years	37	26	46	33	$\chi^2 > 7.82$
12–14 years	18	12	23	15	significant
Never	4	26	5	32	
Total boys	80	80	100	100	

A Commentary

The data on onset age of truanting and stealing can be looked at another way. If those who claimed never to have truanted or stolen are excluded from both groups, then the percentages for onset ages for those who have truanted or stolen in each residual group are as in Table 7.1a.

Thus, although (broadly speaking) truanting delinquents still tend to have started earlier than truanting non-delinquents, no differences in

Table 7.1a: Indications of onset age of truants and stealers

Onset ages	First truanted		First stole	
	Del.	Non-del.	Del.	Non-del.
	%	%	%	%
6–8 years	30	38	28	29
9–11 years	43	19	49	49
12–14 years	27	43	23	22
Totals	100	100	100	100

onset ages appear to occur between delinquents and non-delinquents who steal. (It should be mentioned that the four delinquents who denied ever having stolen were all recidivicts and had been convicted of stealing. Each claimed that he had only 'received' money from others who had stolen it.) It is interesting to find that as many as two-thirds of non-delinquents felt quite free to admit (without any undue pressure on them) that they had previously stolen. (One non-delinquent told the writer in strict confidence that he had just stolen a toy from Woolworth's, and that he still had it in his schoolbag in the classroom. When asked further about this, the boy said that he knew that he was not the only one who would *occasionally* steal things. He believed that he was not doing any real harm because he knew that he would stop stealing immediately if caught by the police or by his parents).

The majority of non-delinquent boys told the writer that their favourite stealing episodes involved stealing fruit from the shops and carts. It was rather obvious that they regarded this merely as a form of game. They usually called this 'scrumping'. Most of the non-delinquents also admitted that they had taken pennies that were said to be lying around in the home. The line between 'scrumping' and more pronounced stealing appeared to be a very narrow one in a considerable number of cases. It was also found that non-delinquents usually smiled cheerfully when relating their stealing episodes, whereas delinquents were tense when discussing such details.

The features which seemed to distinguish most of the delinquents from the non-delinquents were that the non-delinquents kept stressing that (a) they would only *occasionally* steal and (b) that they were scared of being caught by the police or by their parents and maintained that they would stop if they were caught.

7.2 *It is hypothesized that parents of delinquents are less aware of their boys' stealing than those of non-delinquents.*

This hypothesis naturally stems from sub-hypothesis 2.2a in parent-child psychological communication (Chapter 2) that delinquents when in trouble tend *not* to turn to their parents, whereas non-delinquents do turn to their parents.

The Results

Table 7.2 shows that in the cases of three-fifths (60%) of delinquents one or both of their parents were not aware of their boys' stealing; whereas among the bulk (83%) of non-delinquents both parents were aware of their boys' stealing.

Thus the hypothesis was confirmed.

Table 7.2: Indications of parental awareness of their boys' deviant behaviour

Parents aware of boys' deviancy	Numbers		Percentages		
	Del.	Non-del.	Del.	Non-del.	
Both parents One or neither	12 18	25 5	% 40 60	% 83 17	$\chi^2 > 3\cdot84$ significant
Total parents	30	30	100	100	

A Commentary

The author found among both groups of boys that it was the father who was told last about the stealing acts of their boys.

7.3 *It is hypothesized that parents of delinquents tend to show a general inadequacy in dealing with their boys' delinquent activities.*

Clayborne (1954) suggests that parents of delinquents tend to become stricter with their children after they have committed several offences.

However, two other possibilities exist, namely: parents do not change their treatment of the boy (thus seeming incapable of meeting the crisis which is involved in their boy being caught in delinquent acts); or parents become less strict.

The hypothesis was tested by the following questions:
   i. Has your mother become stricter since you first got into trouble?
$$(Q.4.6)$$
   ii. Has your father become stricter since you first got into trouble?
$$(Q.4.7)$$

The Results

Table 7.3 shows that among the bulk of delinquents, both parents did not change their treatment of their boys after the boys got into trouble.

Thus the hypothesis was confirmed.

Table 7.3: Indications of changes in parents' treatment of delinquents after the latter's troubles

Treatment of boy by:	Delinquents	
	Numbers	*Percentages*
Mothers		%
More strict	3	10
The same	27	90
Fathers		
More strict	4	13
Less strict	1	3
The same	25	84
Total	30	100

A Commentary

Clearly Clayborne's suggestion was not substantiated. The hypothesis was substantiated in that in spite of the boys' delinquent behaviour neither parent of most delinquents changed their treatment of their boys (when a change was obviously called for).

Agreement Code

The results of the parent-child agreement code (see Table 7.A below) show incomplete agreement between the answers of the parents and boys among half (47%) of delinquents, and complete agreement between the answers of the parents and boys among the bulk (80%) of delinquents.

Table 7.A: *Agreement code on delinquency*

Parent-child agreement	Numbers		Percentages		
	Del.	Non-del.	Del.	Non-del.	
			%	%	
Complete	16	24	53	80	$\chi^2 > 3 \cdot 84$
Incomplete	14	6	47	20	significant
Total families	30	30	100	100	

Unlike the agreement codes in previous chapters, the above one showed a substantial proportion of incomplete parent-child agreement among the delinquents. Two partial explanations suggest themselves for the parents' answers not lining up with those of their delinquent boys:

i. some parents' ignorance of their boys' delinquency (as shown in Table 7.2);
ii. some of the parents distorted their replies because perhaps they were more ego involved in the topic of delinquency than in the topics of previous chapters, because the latter topics seemed less important to them than the poignant subject of delinquency.

SUMMARY

Summing up this chapter, it can be said:

i. deviant behaviour (i.e. truanting and stealing) was more widespread and tended to start at an earlier age among delinquents than among non-delinquents;
ii. parents of delinquents tended to be less aware of their boys' stealing than did parents of non-delinquents;

iii. parents of delinquents tended to show a general inadequacy in dealing with their boys' delinquent acts.

Section Summary

The findings so far in this study have shown that, as far as the playing of parental roles are concerned, delinquents are differentiated from non-delinquents in the following broad respects:

i. delinquents experience less adequate emotional relationships with their parents (but especially with their fathers);
ii. delinquents experience less adequate training from their parents (but especially from their fathers).

The consequences of the less adequately played roles of the parents of delinquents is manifested by:

i. delinquents having a greater potential for delinquency in that they are more aggressive than non-delinquents in their reactions to stress situations and have probably less constructive extra-familial social contacts;
ii. more widespread deviant behaviour, starting at an earlier age, among delinquents than among non-delinquents.

Again, in relation to the consequences of their role playing, parents of delinquents showed their inadequacies compared with those of non-delinquents in that they were less aware of their boys' deviant behaviour. Even when they became aware of such behaviour, their response was the inadequate one of 'no change'.

Section 4 : Separation

It has been shown in the previous sections that faulty parent-child relationships, especially between the child and the father, seem to be highly correlated with delinquency. This theme is taken up further in this section by focusing the attention on separations which may have occurred between a child and his parents with possible damaging results from the point of view of the child's character formation.

As previously stated, this study deliberately excluded boys from broken homes, the aim being to enable the study of subtle 'under the roof' relationships of the child with *both* parents.

The exclusion of this gross form of parent-child separation did not, however, necessarily eliminate less dramatic (but still vital) forms of parent-child separation from the study.

It is necessary here to distinguish three possible forms of parent-child separation (which are often not clearly enough enunciated), namely:

i. pyschological separation as a concomitant of physical separation (which appears to be the only form usually considered by theorists of 'maternal deprivation');

ii. psychological separation without physical separation;

iii. physical separation without concomitant psychological separation.

This scheme is admittedly a simplification of the issues involved, but it does have useful expository purposes in this section of the study. What follows is not a detailed discussion of the complexities underlying this schema, but merely a few brief points in order to clarify the function of Chapter 8 following.

Firstly, this schema serves to distinguish between psychological separation and physical separation. Some aspects of parent-child psychological separation have been studied in previous chapters (especially Chapter 1 on parental affection and Chapter 2 on parent-child communication) and certain marked differences between delinquents and non-delinquents were found. However, apart from certain features of 'environmental' communication studied in Chapter 2 (e.g. parental leisure time), no attempt has been made so far in this study to see if parent-child physical separations (and any psychological consequences) are important differentiating features between delinquents and non-delinquents. Chapter 8, then, seeks to cover this point.

Secondly, apart from its own intrinsic merits, a study of physical separation between the child and one or both of its parents is of interest in further probing the possible validity of the theory that 'maternal deprivation' is of overriding importance in the aetiology of delinquency. This is so because, although 'maternal deprivation' covers psychological separation whether or not it is due to physical separation, Bowlby and others do place much emphasis on the psychological consequences of physical separation (without necessarily using the distinctions and terminology of the present author).

Thus Chapter 8 performs the functions of studying parent child physical separation as a possible differentiating feature between delinquents and non-delinquents and, consequently, of further partially testing the possible validity of the theory of 'maternal deprivation' (in so far as physical separation is involved).

8 : PHYSICAL SEPARATION

As has been said, the theorists of 'maternal deprivation' tend to concentrate on mother-child psychological separation as a *consequence* of mother-child *physical* separation. This chapter, then concerned as it is with physical separations, is a further partial test of the theory of 'maternal deprivation'. In line with his general approach, the author feels that the latter cannot be tested without reference to the fathers; hence physical separation from both parents will be studied in this chapter. To do this, it is necessary to distinguish (and this is not usually done) three possible forms of parent-child physical separation.

These are:

i. separation of the child from its mother only (or maternal separation);
ii. separation of the child from its father only (or paternal separation);
iii. separation of the child from both of its parents (or dual-parental separation).

The theorists of 'maternal deprivation' naturally, in line with their theory of the primacy of the mothers' role and the secondary nature of the father's role, concentrate on separation of the child from its mother (due to points 'i' and/or 'iii' above) to the exclusion of separation of the child from its father (due to points 'ii' and 'iii' above). Thus they ignore the possible importance of paternal separation and dual-parent separation. The author of the present study, in line with his basic aim of studying the roles of both parents, felt it necessary to study each of the above forms of separation as possible sources of differentiating features between delinquents and non-delinquents.

As was shown in the tripartite schema in the introduction to this section, physical separation does not necessarily involve psychological separation. Hence the author had to devise some criteria for determining whether or not given parent-child physical separations would lead to parent-child psychological separation.

Bowlby has devised criteria of what constitutes possible character damaging due to 'maternal deprivation'. The author of the present study adopted Bowlby's criteria for application to maternal, paternal and dual-parental physical separations. Thus the criteria for possible character damaging parent-child physical separation were:

i. the child's age when separation occurred;
ii. the length of the separation;
iii. the degree of the separation;
iv. the frequency of separation;
v. the quality of parent-child relationships before separation occurred;
vi. the experience of the child with its parent substitute;
vii. the reception the child received from its parents when reunited with them.

As regards the child's age when separation occurred, the author adopted Bowlby's views on what might be termed the 'chronology of vulnerability'. Thus, on this view, damage to the childs' character formation through parent-child separation is potentially greatest if it occurs between the ages of 6 months and 18 months. The child is less vulnerable if aged between 18 months and 3 years and even less so if aged between 3 years and 5 years. Between 5 years and 8 years, the child, although still vulnerable, can survive parent-child separation with considerably less damage to its character development.

Clearly, given the limitations of time and of the recall-questionnaire technique, precise data on all these criteria could not be obtained. However, it was felt that the research tool used (although crude for the task involved) was adequate enough to show whether or not material differences between delinquents and non-delinquents exist in respect of some of these criteria – at least to show whether or not differences applied in respect of fathers as well as mothers.

The author's next task was to determine what sorts of physical separations characterized the three basic forms of parent-child physical separations (i.e. maternal, paternal and dual-paternal). Given the limitations of his research tool, the author decided to study the separation given in the table on page 104.

For each of these types of separation, the attempt was made to determine the child's age at the time of each separation and the length of each separation.

As a side comment on the table, it should be noted that the child's evacuation and the child's hospitalization are often cited as

Selected types of parent-child physical separation characteristic of each of the three basic forms

Maternal separation	Paternal separation	Dual-parental separation
i. Mother working ii. Mother's hospitalization	i. Father's war service ii. Evacuation of the child with its mother iii. Father's shift work, etc. iv. Father's hospitalization	i. Evacuation of the child by itself ii. Child's hospitalization iii. Both parents' hospitalization

instances of 'maternal deprivation'. This is a logical fallacy since the table shows two modes of evacuation of the child (with mother or by itself) associated respectively with paternal and dual-parental separation and child's hospitalization associated with dual-parental separation – i.e. no purely maternal separation involved.

The norm from which the above separations might be considered as potentially character damaging deviations is a peacetime family in which the father does a 'normal' days work (i.e. no excessive overtime work, etc.) and the mother does not work (at least during the child's infancy) and where both parents and children are relatively healthy.

Thus the attempt was made to cover Bowlby's criteria 'i', 'ii' and 'iv' (as stated on page 103). As regards criteria 'v' and 'vii' (qualities of the parent-child relationships respectively before and after physical separation), piloting of relevant questions had shown that only very superficial answers could be obtained by direct questioning. The author relied, therefore, on the questions regarding the basic mother-child and father-child love relationships outlined in Section I (primarily Chapter 1). As regards criteria 'iii' (degree of separation) and 'vi' (the parent substitute) questions were asked about those children who were evacuated by themselves. Because only a fifth (or less) of either group had been evacuated on their own (see Table 8.3) and then, in the main, to relatives (e.g. grandmother or aunt) with whom they stayed rarely for more than a month, the results on the questions were not significant. Further, only two of these cases in each group

could be said to have suffered from a real lack of necessary contact
with their parents (the criteria for 'close contact' being whether or
not parents sent regular letters to the foster-parents, to be read out to
the children and whether or not parents made frequent visits to the
children).

Thus the findings outlined below cover Bowlby's criteria 'i', 'ii'
and 'iv' only, but cover them for mothers *and* fathers.

8.1 *It is hypothesized that there is a greater tendency for delinquents to
have suffered maternal separation than for non-delinquents.*

The reasons for setting up this hypothesis have already been discussed.
Note that the hypothesis is stated in terms of maternal *separation*
and not maternal *deprivation* in keeping with the arguements outlined previously. The hypothesis was tested by the following questions:

   i. How old were you when your mother first started to go out to
      work?   ($Q.2.3$)
  ii. Were there any other separations, apart from evacuation and
      your illnesses, between you and either of your parents (e.g. has
      your mother or your father been ill and had to go to hospital)?
                                            ($Q.5.12$)

It will be noted that the second question ($Q.5.12$) covers an aspect of
each of these basic forms of parent-child separation. Only a few boys
in each group (with no significant differences between the groups)
had experienced separation from either or both parents via parental
hospitalization. Hence the results shown below for this question cover
any parental hospitalization (not only maternal) and will not be
repeated in the results for the two hypotheses respectively on paternal
separation and dual-parental separation.

The Results

Table 8.1 shows:

   i. no significant differences between the two groups as regards the
      age of the boys when their mother first started to work;
  ii. only a negligible proportion of either group appeared to have
      suffered from maternal separation due to parental hospitali-
      zations.

Thus, hypothesis 8.1, that delinquents suffered more from maternal
separation than non-delinquents, was not confirmed.

Table 8.1: *Indications of maternal separation*

	Numbers		Percentages		
	Del.	Non-del.	Del.	Non-del.	
			%	%	
Boy's answers: Age of boy when mother first worked Don't know 0–15 years	58 22	67 13	73 27	84 16	$\chi^2 < 3\cdot84$ not significant
Were parents hospitalized? Yes No	6 74	1 79	7 93	1 99	$\chi^2 < 3\cdot84$ not significant
Total boys	80	80	100	100	
Parents' answers; Age of boy when mother first worked Don't know 0–15 years	19 11	22 8	64 36	73 27	$\chi^2 < 3\cdot84$ not significant
Were parents hospitalized? Yes No	— 30	4 26	— 100	13 87	$\chi^2 < 3\cdot84$ not significant
Total parents	30	30	100	100	

A Commentary

A point that was previously made in this book seems to be worth reiterating here. The fact that a hypothesis was not confirmed does not always mean that it is untrue.

It is quite clear in the case of the age of the boy when the mother first worked that the memory factor (the large proportion of 'don't know') plus the necessity of combining the answers into the all-inclusive age group '0–15 years' (due to statistical requirement of combining cells with less than 5 members) *might* have prevented significant results from emerging.

In the case of parental hospitalization, it required considerable probing to elicit positive answers and the author had to forgo much probing because of the time factor and the dubious value of the results of much probing.

Thus, the results of attempting to test the hypothesis on maternal separation were not strong enough either to refute it or to confirm it.

8.2 *It is hypothesized that there is a greater tendency for delinquents to have suffered paternal separation than for non-delinquents.*

The reasons for setting up this hypothesis have already been discussed. The hypothesis was tested by the following questions:

i. Was your father away during the war? (Q.5.10)
ii. How old were you at the beginning and at the end of his war service? (Q.5.11)
iii. Were you evacuated with your mother during the war? (Q.5.4)
iv. Is your father very often on shift work, or on overtime work, or on work that takes him away from home overnight? (Q.2.6)
v. How old were you when your father was frequently on shift work or away? (Q.2.7)
vi. Were there any other separations, apart from evacuation and your illnesses, between you and either of your parents (e.g. has your mother or your father been ill and had to go to hospital)?. (Q.5.12)

The results for the question (Q.5.12) have already been given under hypothesis 8.1 and will not be repeated here.

The Results

Table 8.2 shows that no significant differences emerged in respect of:

i. fathers' absences from home due to war service;
ii. boys being evacuated with their mothers.

Table 8.2: *Indications of paternal separation*

	Numbers		Percentages		
	Del.	Non-del.	Del.	Non-del.	
			%	%	
Boys' answers: Boys' ages during fathers' war se*vi*ce: 0–6 years Father not absent	36 44	47 33	45 55	59 41	$\chi^2 < 3\cdot84$ not significant
Boy evacuated with his mother Yes No	35 45	28 52	44 56	35 65	$\chi^2 < 3\cdot84$ not significant
Father absent a lot for work reasons when boy was aged: 0–15 (inclusive) Don't know	29 51	25 55	36 64	31 69	$\chi^2 < 3\cdot84$ not significant
Total boys	80	80	100	100	
Parents' answers: Boys' ages during fathers' war service: 0–6 years Father not absent	14 16	18 12	47 53	60 40	$\chi^2 < 3\cdot84$ not significant
Boy evacuated with his mother Yes No	16 14	10 20	53 47	33 67	$\chi^2 < 3\cdot84$ not significant
Father absent a lot for work reasons when boy was aged: 0–15 (inclusive) Don't know	14 16	4 26	47 53	13 87	$\chi^2 > 3\cdot84$ significant
Total parents	30	30	100	100	

However, the parents' answers (which, in respect of early separations, are more reliable than those of the boys) indicate that delinquents suffered more than non-delinquents from paternal separation due to fathers' absence on work duties. However, it was not possible to determine how far such separation applied to the crucial early years, because both parents and boys found it difficult to remember such details.

Thus, hypothesis 8.2, that delinquents suffered more than non-delinquents from paternal separation, cannot be said to have been confirmed. (This is perhaps not surprising if the concept of paternal separation is stretched to that of paternal deprivation analogous to that of maternal deprivation and applied to a criterion such as fathers' damaging absence due to war service. It should be remembered that delinquency has always flourished irrespective of wars.)

A Commentary

Because no significant differences were found between the two groups in respect of separation from the fathers due to the fathers' war service or the boys' evacuation with their mothers and because paternal separation due to work duties could not necessarily be attributed to the earlier years of the boys, it cannot be said that paternal separation with consequent psychological separation is a differentiating feature between delinquents and non-delinquents. Paternal separation in later years due to work duties can, as has been pointed out in Environmental Communication (in Chapter 2), be regarded as a contributory factor to poor father-child communication. But this, although vitally important, is not the same as deprivation in Bowlby's sense.

8.3 *It is hypothesized that there is a greater tendency for delinquents to have suffered from dual-parental separation than for non-delinquents.*
The reasons for setting up this hypothesis have already been stated. The hypothesis was tested by the following questions:

i. Were you evacuated on your own, that is, sent away because of bombing during the war?   (Q.5.2)
ii. How old were you at the beginning and at the end of this evacuation?   (Q.5.3)
iii. Have you had any illnesses which made it necessary for you to go to hospital for more than one week during the first three

years of your life? How old were you, what was the illness, how long did it last, how long were you in hostipal? (*Q.*5.1)

iv. Were there any other separations, apart from evacuation and your illnesses, between you and either of your parents (e.g. has your mother or your father been ill and had to go to hospital)? (*Q.*5.12)

Again, the results for the last question (*Q.*5.12) are not reported below.

Table 8.3: *Indications of parental separation*

	Numbers		Percentages		
	Del.	Non-del.	Del.	Non-del.	
Boys' answers *Boy evacuated by himself*			%	%	
Yes (0–6 years)	15	21	19	26	$\chi^2 < 3\cdot84$
No	65	59	81	74	not significant
Boy hospitalized					
Yes (0–3 years)	16	11	20	14	$\chi^2 < 3\cdot84$
No	64	69	80	86	not significant
Total boys	80	80	100	100	
Parents' answers *Boy evacuated by himself*					
Yes (0–6 years)	6	5	20	17	$\chi^2 < 3\cdot84$
No	24	25	80	83	not significant
Boy hospitalized					
Yes (0–3 years)	6	4	20	13	$\chi^2 < 3\cdot84$
No	24	26	80	87	not significant
Total parents	30	30	100	100	

The Results

Table 8.3 shows no significant differences between delinquents and non-delinquents in respect of dual-parental separation due to:

   i. boys being evacuated by themselves during the war;
  ii. boys being hospitalized when aged under three years.

Thus, hypothesis 8.3, that delinquents suffered more than non-delinquents from dual-parental separation, is not confirmed.

A Commentary

Clearly, greater separation from both parents among delinquents than among non-delinquents was not proven.

Summary and Agreement Codes

No parent-child agreement codes were devised on physical separation because the Tables 8.1 to 8.3 have shown both boys' and parents' answers and indicated no marked disparity to have occurred (except in the case of fathers' absences due to work).

  A summary code has been devised based on answers to questions

Table 8.SC: Summary code on degree of parent-child physical separation

Boy separated	Boys' age at separation	Numbers		Percentages		
		Del.	Non-del.	Del.	Non-del.	
				%	%	
Father	6 months–3 yrs.	12	6	15	8	
Both parents	6 months–3 yrs. or 3 to 6 years	9	8	11	10	
Father and mother	0–6 years ⎱ 0–3 years ⎰	7	13	9	16	$\chi^2 < 11\cdot07$ not significant
Father and mother	0–3 years ⎱ 3–6 years ⎰	11	4	14	5	
Father	0–6 years	29	31	31	39	
Neither parent		12	18	18	22	
Total boys		80	80	100	100	

2.3, 8.10, 8.11, 8.4, 5.2, 5.3 and 5.1. The code merely serves to re-emphasize the difficulties met with in attempting to study differences between the two groups as regards the three basic forms of parent-child physical separation.

SUMMARY

This chapter has attempted to determine whether or not differences exist between delinquents and non-delinquents (who have not suffered from broken homes) as regards three basic forms of parent-child physical separation, namely, maternal (mother only), paternal (father only), and dual-parental (both mother and father).

The study of such physical separations is important in its own right, but also serves as a further test of the possible validity of the theory that 'maternal deprivation' is an all-important factor in the aetiology of delinquency. The latter test is important because in the theory of 'maternal deprivation' physical separation would appear to be a most (if not *the* most) important cause of psychological separation between mother and child (the latter occurring during and/or after physical separation). Because the 'maternal deprivation' theory assumes that any negative father-child relationships that might occur are preceded by and (hence) are *secondary* to negative mother-child relationships (e.g. Friendlander, 1947), the theory considers physical separations only in so far as the mother is involved and often tends to ignore the fact that the father might also importantly be involved in some of these mother-child separations (i.e. dual-parental separation) and ignores other separations where the mother is not involved (i.e. paternal separation).

Because of his general aim of examining the roles of both parents, the present author did not feel able unconditionally to accept the assumptions and consequent emphasis of the 'maternal deprivation' theory. This led him to distinguish three possible forms of parent-child physical separation (and some types of physical separation associated with each form) and to investigate which, if any, servd to distinguish delinquents from non-delinquents.

The findings of this chapter show, with one exception, no significant distinctions between delinquents and non-delinquents on the three forms of parent-child physical separation. The exception was the case of paternal separation due to work duties, but this finding was reduced in value because the boys' ages at which separation occurred could not be obtained with any precision. The most that can be said is that the tendency of fathers of delinquents to have greater work demands leads to less communication with their boys than is the case with fathers of non-delinquents.

Another limitation of the findings was that it was not possible to distinguish whether or not individual physical separations give rise to psychological separation. Thus, even if some parent-child physical separations had been found to differentiate between delinquents and non-delinquents, it could not necessarily be assumed that these had caused psychological separation (since physical separation does not necessarily involve psychological separation). Basically, then, the findings lead one to conclude that the recall-questionnaire technique (or, indeed, any retrospective study technique) is too blunt a research tool to show up causative links between physical separation and psychological separation – at least, where broken homes are not involved. This is because the use of such a technique does not obtain sound data on all the criteria which determine whether or not physical separation might have involved psychological separation.

Thus the findings could neither validate nor invalidate the theory of 'maternal deprivation'. However, they do call the general usefulness of this theory into question. The reasoning behind this assertion is as follows:

i. to be of heuristic value, a theory must incorporate clearly defined empirical referents and must be susceptible to empirical testing by a *practical* research method operating on these re-referents;

ii. apart from the fact that the 'maternal deprivation' theory does not satisfactorily provide clearly defined empirical referents, it is not, in certain crucial respects, susceptible to empirical testing by a *practical* research method (as the findings in this chapter testify).

It might be claimed that the theory of 'maternal deprivation' could be empirically tested by research methods other than a cross-sectional retrospective technique (which, incidentally, is the technique primarily used by theorists of 'maternal deprivation').

In theory this is true, and the technique involved would have to be longitudinal studies of children from birth to early 'teens in a representative sample of families. However, the sample would have to be large in order to ensure that a statistically adequate number of delinquents would emerge in the sample, and the study would have to be on the roles of *both* parents – not merely on those of mothers. This would be a recognition of the principle that apart from sibling relationships, a basic family structure consists of a triangle of subtle relationships between mother, father and child which condition the degree of mental health (or ill health) of the child.

Part Three

CONCLUSIONS

1 : SUMMARY OF THE STUDY

INTRODUCTION

The object of this chapter is to summarize this empirical study of perception of parental roles and their relevance to differentiating between delinquents and non-delinquents. The summary is divided into three parts, namely:

i. Objects of the Study – which briefly restates the primary objects in carrying out this study.
ii. Technique – which briefly restates the key features of how the the study was carried out.
iii. The Findings – which briefly summarizes the main findings of the study.

A fuller discussion of the theoretical and practical implications of this study is left to the next chapter (Conclusions).

The main objects of this study were:

i. to reinvestigate thoroughly the roles of *both* parents in order to determine whether differences exist between delinquents and non-delinquents in regard to the adequacy with which each parent plays his/her role;
ii. To measure this adequacy mainly in terms of the child's perception of the roles played by its parents and also in terms of the parents' perceptions of their own roles;
iii. to develop a research tool of practical diagnostic value to clinicians working in those child-guidance centres dealing mainly with juvenile delinquents and their parents.

TECHNIQUE

In essence, the technique used in this study was personal individual interviewing (conducted by means of a formal interview-questionnaire) of a test sample of delinquents boy and a control sample of non-delinquent boys. The need for a control group is obviously necessary if the study was to highlight uniquely delinquent traits. Without a control group there would be no means of knowing which revealed

119

traits were uniquely delinquent and which were common to both delinquents and non-delinquents.

The Samples

Each sample consisted of 80 boys, and group-matching of the samples was made in respect of the following characteristics:

  i. geographical location – confined to London 'delinquency areas';
 ii. age of boys – confined to those aged 12–15 years;
iii. intelligence quotient – confined to those with I.Q.s between 80 and 125 (thus excluding mental defectives);
 iv. mental state – confined to non-neurotics and non-psychopaths;
  v. socio-economic characteristics – confined to boys from working-class homes (from whence the bulk of delinquents come);
 vi. family background – confined to boys from unbroken homes.

The delinquent samples consisted solely of recidivist thieves (rare cases, such as sex offenders and incendiarists, were excluded from the sample) from a Remand Home. The non-delinquents sample consisted of boys from two adjacent Secondary Modern Schools.

In each sample a sub-sample of 30 boys was selected and both their parents interviewed.

The Questionnaire

The questionnaire was designed to test a series of hypotheses covering a number of wide areas of the boys' life experiences (primarily of the boys' perceptions of their parents' roles). The same questionnaire with necessary modifications of phrasing was used on the parents of the two sub-samples of 30 boys.

The Fieldwork

The fieldwork was carried out as follows:

  i. all delinquent boys, and the parents of the 30 boys in the sub-sample, were interviewed at the Remand Home;
 ii. all non-delinquent boys were interviewed at their respective schools and the parents of the 30 boys in the sub-sample were interviewed at their homes.

Analysis of the Results

The results from the 80 boys in each sample were subjected to tests for significant inter-sample differences by means of the Chi-square test at the 5% level of confidence. The results from certain questions in each area of life covered by the questionnaire were cross-analysed to give a summary code for the given area – which summarized the main findings of the area. The answers of the parents of each of the two sub-samples of 30 boys were cross-analysed with those of the boys in the sub-samples to give parent-child agreement codes – which indicated the degree of agreement between the answers of the parents and boys.

Summing-up

Thus, given the admitted limitations of the cross-sectional recall method by an individual interviewer, every endeavour was made to ensure an adequate test design and thereby to minimize the limitations.

THE FINDINGS

The findings will be summarized chapter by chapter, under the relevant section and chapter headings.

Section I: The Emotional Atmosphere

The first three chapters studied aspects of parent-child emotional relationships. Such relationships were felt to be both general condition, and an active determinent of other aspects of the child's general training in the process of socialization.

Chapter 1 – *Parental Affection:*

This chapter was concerned with certain aspects of the general parent-child affective relationships. This chapter was central to the whole study in that sound parent-child love relationships are a basic pre-condition and active determinant of the adequacy of parental role playing. The chapter also represented in some ways a test of the equivocal theory that 'maternal deprivation' is mostly the primary factor in the aetiology of delinquency.

The findings were that:

  i. delinquents tended to feel that their mother loved them most, whereas non-delinquents tended to feel loved by both parents – thus the differentiating feature here was the inadequate love given by the father among delinquents;
 ii. delinquents tended to feel that their parents (but especially

    their fathers) were embarrassed to show open affection for them, whereas non-delinquents did not feel this;

iii. delinquents tended more than non-delinquents to feel embarrassed at showing open love for their parents – implying a casual linking with 'ii' above;

iv. delinquents tended to feel 'nagged' by their parents, whereas non-delinquents did not feel this;

v. delinquents tended to feel they had their mothers' *ways* rather than their fathers' *ways*, whereas non-delinquents tended to feel they had both parents' ways or their fathers' *ways* – thus indicating that delinquents tend less to identify with their fathers than do non-delinquents.

Thus, compared with non-delinquents, delinquents receive less strong and open love from their parents – but especially in the case of their fathers. Such a finding, although not denying the importance of mothers' roles, is not consistent with the theory that 'maternal deprivation' is the *main* aetiological factor in delinquency – at least as far as boys from this sample are concerned.

Chapter 2 – Parent-child Communication

Two interacting aspects of parent-child communication were distinguished, namely, environmental and psychological.

    The findings on environmental communication were:

i. fathers of delinquents tended to have less leisure time available (due allegedly to work duties) for contacts with their children than did fathers of non-delinquents (there were no significant differences between the groups as far as mothers were concerned);

ii. the quantity of leisure-time contacts between parents and child was much lower among delinquents than among non-delinquents;

iii. the quality of leisure-time contacts between parents and child was much lower among delinquents than among non-delinquents – this was definitely established as regards fathers of delinquents (less father-child sharing of hobbies and outings);

iv. that it was the fathers rather than the mothers of delinquents who were regarded as being most deficient in environmental communication, was indicated by the fact that the bulk of delinquents felt that it would be helpful if they could see more of their fathers, but the majority did not feel this about their mothers (the bulk of non-delinquents did not feel a need to see more of either parent).

In short, both parents of delinquents were viewed as inadequate by the boys in environmental communication, whereas both parents of non-delinquents were viewed as adequate. However, there were very strong indications that it was the fathers' defective roles that most troubled delinquents – which seems only natural since one would expect that a boy would desire positive leisure time contacts more with his father than with his mother.

The findings on psychological communication were that:

i. the bulk of delinquents tended not to contact their parents when in trouble, whereas the bulk of non-delinquents did so;
ii. delinquents tended to prefer their mothers to deal ultimately with their wrongdoings, whereas non-delinquents tended to prefer their fathers to do so;
iii. delinquents tended to turn to their mothers for general advice, whereas non-delinquents tended to turn to their fathers or both parents.

As regards which parent was felt to understand the boy most and which parent the boy turned to *initially* when in trouble, both groups gave a clear preference for their mothers – which means that these items do not differentiate between the two groups.

Briefly, then, the fathers' psychological communication was viewed as inadequate among delinquents, whereas both parents were viewed as adequate among non-delinquents.

Chapter 3 – Home Climate

This chapter was a study of some heterogeneous factors that rounded off the section on the 'emotional atmosphere'. The findings were that, superficially, the home atmosphere, as measured by perceived parental quarrelling, did not appear to differ as between delinquents and non-delinquents. However, two features were indicative of greater home tensions among delinquents, namely:

i. fathers of delinquents contributed towards general tension by appearing to be less cheerful in the home;
ii. inter-sibling quarrels were more rife in homes of delinquents.

Thus, summing up the section on the emotional atmosphere, delinquents experienced, in general, inadequate and tense emotional relationships with their fathers, but to a lesser extent with their mothers, whereas non-delinquents experienced, in general, adequate emotional relationships with both parents.

Section II: Training

The next two chapters were concerned with studying two stages of parental training of the child, namely, training in infancy (by the mother) and training in later years (by both parents).

Chapter 4 – Infant Training

The findings of this chapter were that:

  i. no significant differences existed between delinquents and non-delinquents as regards infant maturation in bowel training, bladder training, sitting up, cutting teeth, walking, talking;
 ii. delinquents tended to have been breast-fed for shorter periods than non-delinquents.

Thus, basically, no material differences in infant training were found between delinquents and non-delinquents.

Chapter 5 – Later Training

The findings of this chapter were:

  i. among delinquents there was a tendency for their fathers not to appear clearly as the effective leader of the family, whereas among non-delinquents their fathers clearly appeared as effective leaders of the family;
 ii. among delinquents there was a greater tendency for fathers rather than mothers to display over-emotional reactions to trouble than was the case with non-delinquents;
iii. among non-delinquents there was a slightly greater tendency for parents to show 'reasonableness' in meting out punishments than among delinquents (fathers of delinquents being more implicated here);
 iv. among delinquents there was a very marked tendency for parents not to strike the right balance as regards strictness (mothers in particular tending towards leniency), whereas among non-delinquents the bulk of parents did strike the right balance;

v. delinquents strongly tended to feel that they should receive more praise from both parents (but especially the father), whereas non-delinquents strongly tended to feel that they received enough praise.

Thus against a background of inadequate and tense emotional relationships with their fathers (as shown by Section I), it was found that delinquents suffered from inadequate later (post-infancy) training from their parents, especially from their fathers.

Section III: Consequences

The next two chapters studied the consequences of the manner in which parental roles were played in terms of the social behaviour of the boys.

Chapter 6 – Dynamics

This chapter studied aspects of the boys' behaviour which, although not specifically delinquent, might indicate whether or not a potentiality for delinquency existed.

The findings of this chapter were:

i. delinquents tended more than non-delinquents to be aggressive in their reaction to stress situations, as shown by their own admitted tendencies to feel anger when they come up against something they do not like:

ii. in line with 'i' above, delinquents tended more than non-delinquents to resent parental punishments;

iii. delinquents tended no more than non-delinquents to copy their fathers' reactions to stress situations;

iv. while delinquents did not appear to be much more prone to social isolation than non-delinquents, it does appear that their outside social activities were probably not as constructive of those of non-delinquents.

Thus, in terms of their aggressive reactions to stress situations and their probable lower quality of outside activities, delinquents display their greater potentiality for delinquency.

Chapter 7 – Delinquency

This chapter studied the boys' more specifically delinquent behaviour and their parents' awareness of and reactions to such behaviour.

The findings were:

   i. deviant behaviour (i.e. truanting and stealing) was more wide-spread and tended to start at an earlier age among delinquents than among non-delinquents;

   ii. parents of delinquents tended to be less aware of their boys' stealing than did parents of non-delinquents;

   iii. parents of delinquents tended to show a general inadequacy in dealing with the delinquent acts of their boys.

Section IV: Separation

This chapter dealt with various forms of parent-child separations. It was pointed out that, although boys from broken homes (the gross form of parent-child separation) had been excluded from study, the possibility remained that less gross forms of separation might have occurred to boys included in the study. Three possible forms of parent-child separation were distinguished, namely:

   i. psychological separation as a concomitant of physical separation;

   ii. psychological separation without physical separation;

   iii. physical separation without concomitant psychological separation.

The theorists of 'maternal deprivation' appear usually to consider the first of the above possible forms. The study of parent-child physical separation, then, was necessary because it had not so far been dealt with in the study and to deal with it would constitute a further partial test of the possible validity of the theory of 'maternal deprivation' (where physical separation is usually given a major role in causing psychological separation between mother and child).

Chapter 8 – Physical Separation

Three basic forms of parent-child physical separation were distinguished and studied, namely, maternal separation, paternal separation and dual-parental separation. It was pointed out that these crucial distinctions were not made by theorists of 'maternal deprivation' because of their disposition to consider the fathers' roles as secondary to those of mothers. Seven criteria were defined determining whether or not given parent-child physical separations would lead to parent-child psychological separation and to a consequent possibility of damage to the child's character formation. However, in the event findings could be shown for only three of these criteria (namely, child's age during separation, length of separation, and frequency of separation). These were applied to certain types of parent-child physical separations associated respectively with each of the three basic forms named above.

The findings of this chapter were:

i. no material differences emerged between delinquents and non-delinquents as regards maternal separations – measured by age of boys when mothers first worked and by whether or not parents were hospitalized;

ii. apart from a greater tendency among delinquents than non-delinquents for their fathers to be away from home (allegedly) due to work duties, no material differences emerged between the two groups as regards the paternal separations – measured by whether or not fathers were absent on war service or boys were evacuated with mothers;

iii. no material differences emerged between the two groups with regards dual-parental separations – measured by whether or not boys were evacuated by themselves or were hospitalized.

It was pointed out that, using the technique of recall questionnaires, it was extremely difficult to get sound data on all the criteria for all the types of separations within each basic form of parent-child physical separation. Hence, as regards the relation of the findings to the theory that 'maternal deprivation' is the primary aetiological factor in delinquency, it was a case of 'not proven' (rather than an invalidation of the theory). It was pointed out that the lack of clearly defined empirical referents in the theory of 'maternal deprivation' and (in any case) the difficulty of framing practical empirical research to test such referents led to the conclusion that the theory of 'maternal deprivation' is of dubious heuristic value as far as differentiating delinquents from non-delinquents is concerned. Whatever research was used would have to study the roles of *both* parents and not merely those of the mother for the research to be of use in testing the validity of the 'maternal deprivation' theory.

Summing Up

Summing up the findings of the study in so far as they involve differences between delinquents and non-delinquents in parental roles (as perceived by the boys and by the parents) it can be said that compared with non-delinquents:

i. delinquents experience less open and strong love from their parents (especially from their fathers);
ii. delinquents experience less adequate communication (both environmental and psychological) with their parents (especially with their fathers);
iii. delinquents experience a more tense home atmosphere (to which their fathers contribute a substantial share);
iv. delinquents experience less adequate parental training (especially from their fathers);
v. the deviant behaviour of delinquents was less known to and less adequately dealt with by their parents.

As regards the three basic forms of physical separation, sound data did not emerge. What data did emerge reinforced the findings on the inadequate roles of fathers of delinquents regarding environmental communication. In all these differences, then, it was the inadequacies in their fathers' roles rather more than in their mothers' roles that served to differentiate delinquents from non-delinquents. These findings completely justified the author's feeling of the necessity to study the roles of *both* parents in that the findings brought out the importance of the (much neglected) roles of fathers in the aetiology of delinquency.

2 : CONCLUSIONS

Most previous studies have concentrated on the role of the mother and its reference to the aetiology of delinquency; in contrast, the present study has examined the roles of both mothers and fathers. This latter procedure was adopted because it was felt that the possible importance of the father's role in the aetiology of delinquency had been very much ignored, and because it was felt that the assertion of the absolute supremacy of the mother's role in the aetiology of delinquency was premature without sufficient examination of the father's role.

The study also departed from previous studies in its emphasis on studying parental roles *as perceived by the boys* and in its investigation of *both the parents' perception of their own roles* (and of the degree of agreement between boys and both parents).

Clearly, the assumption behind the concept of 'role perception' is that, whether or not the *actual* roles of one or both parents highly correlate with the boys' *perception* of them, if the delinquent boys' perceptions of their parents' roles are highly negative and the non-delinquent boys' perceptions positive, then a study of boys' perceptions of parental roles enables delinquents to be distinguished from non-delinquents.

Very briefly, one can conclude from this study that delinquent boys (suffering neither from mental defects or diseases, nor from broken homes) tend to perceive greater defects in their fathers' roles than in their mothers' roles, whereas non-delinquents tend to perceive the roles of both parents as being adequate. (Further, this seems confirmed in the main by both parents). Thus the prime differentiating feature between delinquents and non-delinquents, as far as parental role playing is concerned, is the delinquents' perception of their fathers' role as being negative.

This finding, without denying the importance of the mother's role in the aetiology of delinquency, does, for the type of delinquent examined, tend to deny the absolute supremacy of the mother's role. Inevitably, this conflicts with the basic emphasis of the theory of 'maternal deprivation' – at least, in so far as the latter claims universal validity. Assuming that mother-child relationships are tolerably satisfactory (without, of course, denying the importance of the role during a child's infancy), the factor which may well make the major difference between malformation of character in a child and good mental health may be the extent to which father-child relationships have or have not been established satisfactorily.

This finding in the present study is not very surprising in view of the fact that Freudians have always attached great significance to the Oedipus complex and father figures in super-ego formation. It is, therefore, much less surprising to find in this study that father figures have emerged as being of utmost importance than it is to find in this field that the role of fathers has not been stressed more fully by Freudians themselves. The findings presented in this work are also meaningful if viewed quite apart from a Freudian interpretation and are viewed from the point of view of Learning-Theory and behaviourism. It is understandable that a growing child who has not been grossly deprived of his mother's affection feels entitled to receive at least an equal amount of affection from his father – in other words from both parents equally. If paternal affection towards the child is lacking, ill balance in the family structure must result. Under such circumstances it might be found, for instance, that the mother may try to compensate and unduly to protect the child from the non-loving father. Thus, a child who perceives his father in a negative way over a period of years may gradually not only develop hostility towards the father but may also at a given time start to project such hostility beyond the family scene on to the world at large. Some delinquent acts would seem to be meaningful if interpreted in this light.

The writer has found that a child may perceive his father as being *unsatisfactory* not only in the primary and most important area of affection, but in the majority of 'secondary' areas which involve father-child relationships – such as training, discipline, intercommunication, etc. Conversely, results presented here also tend to be meaningful if one bears in mind the importance of the child's perception of the role of the father as *satisfactory*. A well-adjusted boy seems one who has identified himself with a positive father figure, namely, a wise and loving father who has positive valence in a variety of areas as regards father-child relationships. Where a father shows deficiency primarily in the area of affection and additionally in the other areas, it would seem to be very difficult for a boy to identify himself positively with his father. It is likely that a major conflict may ultimately result which the boy feels compelled to act out negatively outside in society. He cannot or does not want to act out these conflicts inside the home where he views his father as unsatisfactory or as the person who can still be appeased and indirectly appealed to by the very committing of misdemeanours. Juvenile delinquency among boys might, therefore, be regarded in one way as a battle ground where relationships are often fought out primarily between members of the same sex, that is, between a boy and his father or between a boy and figures of authority in society. This interpretation of delinquent acts is, however, relevant only when the boy and his mother enjoy at least some measure of a harmonious relationship. The findings presented in this study are not in conflict with such a theory.

It is now necessary to point out some of the limitations of the present study. Firstly, only a restricted type of delinquent (and non-delinquent) was studied. For a further delineation of parental roles and their consequences, it would be necessary to include, for instance, more advanced delinquents (Borstal boys) and different types of offenders, and use matched samples of delinquents and non-delinquents from both broken and non-broken homes, from all social classes, from other areas of the country, with more varied mental make-ups (e.g. including neurotics). Reasons have been given for the restrictions imposed in this study, but the limitations due to such restrictions remain. Secondly, the sample sizes (of both groups) were small. For the findings of the present study to be fully validated would require a repeat study on much larger samples – especially if some or all of the restrictions mentioned above were to be lifted. In fact, the present study is a pilot study – but one that does have the virtue of being repeatable.

Thirdly, the study is essentially a statistical study of correlations between delinquency and certain features of parental roles. As such it does draw attention to various factors of *possible* aetiological significance involved, but it cannot *prove* them to be such. However, even this limiting feature has positive aspects in that:

i. it gives very strong indications of possible causal factors (and their inter-linking) which it would be worth while to research into further;

ii. the very correlations in themselves, if substantiated by repeating of the study, would indicate that the interview questionnaire has some predictive value and hence is worth while developing as a clinical tool for use in child guidance clinics.

Had the samples been larger, extensive use of factor analysis would have been made in order to isolate more clearly the underlying possible aetiological factors.

Fourthly, the study was chiefly confined to the study of parental roles to the exclusion of other possible delinquency-making factors. The author feels that the time has come for much larger scale and more rigorous research into the causes of delinquency. Such research should be marked by the following characteristics:

   i. the research should be the co-ordinated work of a large team of specialists from many fields of social studies – an inter-disciplinary approach;

  ii. large matched nationally representative samples of delinquents and non-delinquents (as test and control groups respectively) should be used in the research;

 iii. full use should be made of available statistical techniques in the sample design and selection and in analysing the data (e.g. use of computer machines for complex factor analysis);

 iv. the research should be designed to test clearly delineated hypotheses and to arrive at an empirically based theoretical model with high predictive powers.

The opportunity should be taken to extend such research to delinquency among girls.

To sum up the results of the present study, the author feels that they provide strong indications:

   i. that the role of fathers is of great significance in the aetiology of delinquency and that the supremacy of the role of mothers (as claimed by the theory of 'maternal deprivation') is questionable as a universal feature;

  ii. that the research design used was generally adequate for its task;

 iii. that the interview-questionnaire would be worth while developing into a clinical tool;

 iv. that, given the indicated importance of the father's role to a child's development, clinics for the guidance of *both* parents of delinquents and 'problem' children should be set up.

In conclusion, the author hopes to have demonstrated the need for conducting further research into various aspect of juvenile delinquency via an empirical approach of not only studying the child's perception of the role of both parents but also by a concomitant study of the parents' confirmation of their own role playing. Whilst not claiming that this has been done exhaustively in this book, it is hoped that at least a start has been made here in this particular direction.

Appendices

1 : A REVIEW OF THE LITERATURE

The appendix is a brief review of the literature on juvenile delinquency and serves to provide the background against which the author's study has been set. This review excludes the three books covered in Part One, Chapter 1, of this study.

This chapter is divided into five sub-sections, namely:

i. a review of literature concerned with the general background of juvenile delinquency;
ii. a review of literature concerned with parent-child relationships, particularly of 'affection';
iii. a review of literature concerned with constitutional factors;
iv. a review of literature concerned with training problems;
v. a review of literature concerned with communication and group dynamic problems.

GENERAL BACKGROUND STUDIES AND REVIEW OF THE LITERATURE

One of the earliest landmarks in the field of active research in delinquency is the work done by the American, Healy (1915, 1925), who, as early as 1909, set up the 'Juvenile Psychopathic Institute'. The aims of this Institute, the first of its kind, were to assist juvenile courts, to provide a clinical service and, furthermore, to test aetiological hypotheses regarding delinquency. Healy stressed the importance of 'antecedent prior conditions' in the study of delinquency and formulated hypotheses which to this day, though somewhat modified, are held to be true to most workers in the field (for example, the causative factors of defective heredity, broken homes, poor parental control, bad companionship, etc.).

In England, Sir Cyril Burt (1925, 1925a) published his monumental work *The Delinquent* in 1925 which tested many theories which were held to be true in the U.S. and in Great Britain and contained much statistical data on the subject of juvenile delinquency. Burt, like Healy, stressed the aetiological importance of the 'family drama' (i.e. tensions occurring in the family structure) and of early detection of delinquent behaviour. He also advocated the early treatment of offenders.

The years which followed the First World War were to some extent characterized by studies which were related to Freudian theories such as the works of Aichhorn (1936), Steckel (1925), Reich (1925), and, later, Alexander and Staub (1931). These studies, while informative, are based on theories which do not readily lend themselves to statistical validation and must therefore be judged primarily on their qualitative descriptive material. Two studies which deserve specific mention are that of Aichhorn (1936) and Anton Makarenko (1936) (the latter a non-Freudian) whose works have made a contribution to the understanding of psychopathic juveniles. Both of the works referred to observations carried out on groups of young psychopaths. Especially during the decade preceding the Second World War, other researches investigated particular aspects of Freudian theory. For instance, Childers and Hamil (1932) and Goldman (1948) did research on children's feeding habits and the relation between faulty feeding habits and maladjustment.

By 1935 enough research had been carried out to cause authors such as Silverman (1935) to assert with some authority that the aetiological concept of 'a broken home' was useful, but insufficient to explain abnormal behaviour such as neuroticism and delinquency. The concepts of 'a broken home' are apt to mask the many subtle relationships that may exist in a home which though technically 'not broken' is full of internal conflicts existing between various members of the family.

Bennett (1951 and 1960), in a review of the literature in this field, points out clearly that by 1935 considerable agreement had been reached by research workers about the following points:

i. Regarding the causes of delinquency, only theories could be seriously considered which were based on multiple causality and not on single causality.
ii. Inborn constitutional factors seemed less important, other things being equal, than delinquency-fostering family milieux.
iii. Delinquents tended towards low I.Q. and especially educational sub-normality. (This finding has been confirmed by Rose (1949) in his study on delinquents where he found that the mean I.Q. of his cases fell into the 'dull average' group. However, the factor of inherited low intelligence is considered by

most workers to be much less important as a factor in delinquency than faulty inter-family relationships.)

iv Concepts such as guilt, aggression, hostility, insecurity, rejection, frustration, etc., could best be viewed as a result of 'scarred' personality structure rather than the result of inborn mental disease.

v. Child-development studies, in order to yield the maximum amount of information, would have to be closely linked with studies in allied fields to psychology such as jurisprudence, economics, sociology, education, social anthropology.

vi. The study of juvenile delinquency is specialized and distinct from that of neuroticism and also distinct from the study of neurotics who are suffering from delinquency.

vii. Better methods were required to progress from a microscopic approach to one of microscopic specificity.

Whilst during the 1930's the bulk of research work concentrated on home background and family structure, Clifford Shaw (1929, 1938), and later he and his collaborator McKay (1931, 1942) and more recently Morris (1957), stressed the importance of so-called 'delinquency areas' in giving rise to delinquency. These findings indicated that certain geographical areas were more delinquency-producing than others, especially heavily industrialized areas. Studies of this kind left unsolved the problem as to why a high percentage of people coming from so-called delinquency areas failed to become delinquent – a problem which was taken up again by Professor Sprott (1952) who reports that delinquency streets not delinquency areas may well have to be investigated further as causative factors in delinquency. Mannheim (1949), referring to Shaw's study, pointed out that it should be regarded as an ecological and not psychological study in that it concerned itself with habits, modes of life and relations to one's environment. Carr-Saunders, Mannheim and Rhodes (1942), Mannheim (1948) examined a series of hypotheses and in their findings, unlike Shaw, stressed the importance of inter-action between heredity and environment.

During the late 1930s and early 1940s many studies were produced which concentrated more specifically on particular aspects of personality and character development. A series of studies on rejected children was made. One of the best known is that of Levy (1937, 1943), a psycho-analyst who saw certain causal connections in 20 cases between 'primary affect hunger' and 'rejected children'. Other writers on the subject were Bender and Schilder (1937), Zilburg (1937), Menniger (1930), Glover (1933), Rosenhaim (1942), and Lippman (1937, 1945).

Three studies of general interest in this field are that of Linder (1946), who deals with the topic of psychopathy, and of W. F. Whyte (1943), who made a study of group and 'Street Corner Society', and recently that of J. B. Mays (1955) on 'Growing up in a City' (1971), and even more recently gang behaviour has been studied by M. R. de Yarrow, L. Leeuw, and P. Scott (1962), M. R. de Yarrow and M. S. Goodwin (1963), and D. M. Downes (1966).

Of special interest are two authors who emphasize the importance of both mothers and fathers in psychological adjustment of children. Newell (1934, 1936), in tracing the psychodynamics of maternal rejection, found that parents who rejected their children were themselves often maladjusted or emotionally unstable. Mothers who were found to be over-protective or overtly hostile often induced aggression in their children. Another author, Macdonald (1938), is of particular relevance to this thesis since he writes about the relationships between fathers and their children – a topic which is much neglected by researchers in the field. He found in his study that very few delinquent boys had satisfactory relationships with their fathers or a father substitute and that these children had usually been in the complete charge of females who were aggressive, dominant, punitive women. These women were inclined to despise men and feel superior to them. Concurrently, the fathers were inclined to be submissive and depressed persons, unwilling to or incapable of asserting their authority. The problems of aggressive behaviour and various forms of aggression was investigated by Slavson (1943) and the problems of truanting and absconding (two well-known syndromes often associated with delinquency) were investigated by Riemer (1940) and Andriola (1946). The former reports that children who are inclined to run away from either school or home demonstrate a complexity of behavioral symptoms consisting of the following:

i. a feeling of not being loved;
ii. a hurt self-esteem;
iii. resultant aggressive hostility.

Andriola (1946), in an attempt to describe and isolate truancy as a syndrome, concludes that a child who truants (1) has suffered severe parental rejection, especially from his mother, (2) comes from a home where marital disharmony predominates and (3) removes himself from the field because he feels worthless despite the fact that he may be quite intelligent. The field has also recently been studied by, among others, M. B. Clyne (1966).

Apart from specialized research on truanting. other research has been conducted on the origin of enuresis, a symptom which according to Goodman and Michaelis (1934), Karpman (1948) and others, is said to occur frequently in delinquents as well as in neurotics. Michaelis (1938), in studying 100 delinquents and 100 neurotics, presents sound evidence that enuresis and delinquency are in no way causally connected but are themselves the outcome of personality weakness. Alexander and Staub (1931) claim that enuresis is instinctual in the psycho-analytical sense while Mowrer and Mowrer (1938) ascribed enuresis to faulty habit training, and claim that the habit is closely associated with aggression and masturbation.

In recent years interest has returned to the study of inter-family relationships as is shown in Healy and Bronner's well-known studies (1936) and Rutter (1966). As early as 1936 Lowry (1936) described the damage to a child who received too much adoration from his parents. Levy (1943) further developed his own ideas in which he describes various types of over-protective mothers and the effects of over-protection on a child. Bannister and Ravden (1944), by comparing the home environment of normal and problem children, have stressed the importance of discipline in satisfactory adjustment as a factor distinct from that of overprotection. Karpman (1948) agrees essentially with Levy (1943) that maternal over-protection allows the child more instinctual expression; while parental rejection heightens the child's aggressiveness which in turn may lead to delinquent behaviour.

As can be readily seen, by 1940 there was a need to investigate more specific aspects of home background factors. Bowlby (1944, 1946), in studying 44 juvenile thieves, describes a special kind of delinquent known as 'the affectionless character'; and later Bowlby investigated a factor with which his name has become closely connected, namely 'maternal deprivation' – a psychological result of prolonged separation between mother and child. His findings and others on maternal deprivation were further elaborated on and summarized in the well-known World Health Organization Monograph (1952). The ill effects of maternal deprivation have been discussed by several psychoanalysts such as Fenichel (1934, 1945) and Burlingham and Anna Freud (1942, 1943). The latter researchers have published a study on children who were evacuated during World War II and consequently were deprived of their mothers' affection. The authors report that this maternal deprivation caused great psychological damage to the children in that normal character formation was hindered.

The question of character formation is of course crucial to the whole topic so far discussed in this chapter. It is now largely accepted that faulty family background relationships are one of the important factors generally connected with abnormal behaviour (neurotic psychotic and delinquent), but there is not enough evidence to support the theory that it is the *main* cause of maladjustment, nor is there a universally accepted theory which explains how faulty family relationships harm the child. One hypothesis is that faulty family background relationships are harmful because they hinder healthy character development and prevent adequate formation of a conscience. The concept of conscience has exercised the minds of many philosophers, metaphysicians, and recently psychologists; and many hypothetical constructs have been suggested to explain the phenomenon. MacDougall (1908), according to his theory of instincts, traced several stages in the development of the conscience. Freud (1914, 1917), in his papers on narcissism and mourning and melancholia, summarized his views on conscience and character formation. These are quoted as follows: 'Conscience formation proceeds by way of repeated partial identification with a loved person which usually occurs after temporary withdrawal of love from that person following frustration of instinctual urges in the ordinary course of education. The identification results in a change in the ego in order to resemble the loved person; in a sense the child obtains his independence at a price, he introjects the parents' demands in order to be free of them and of other controls.' Bennett (1952) refers to Freud's works in which he points out that the strength of the conscience is directly dependent upon the strength and number of the early love relationships between the child and the parents, and that a weakening of the earliest emotional ties is reflected in a corresponding weakness in the super-ego or conscience. Frequently, it is not the loss but the psychological withdrawal of the loved person which leads to a lack of identification with that person. In delinquents the love relationship between child and parents is progressively weakened. The result is a lack of identification with the parent and abnormal character formation. In this connection, Bowlby states that loss of maternal love, if experienced frequently and deeply by a child between the age of 6–18 months, produces a condition in the child which makes normal attachments increasingly difficult (Bowlby 1952). Healthy growth would seem to be largely dependent on constant and gradual long-term conflicts – the repetition of the pattern of loving, frustration withdrawal identification – which normally leads to fundamental changes in the character based upon strong and well-knit identification with the parents and other parent surrogate figures.

It must be remembered that a number of theories (including that of Melaine Klein) are now in existence which are in opposition to the Freudian hypothesis of character formation. Some of these other theories, as well as the Freudian concepts, are in need of being validated. Non-Freudian theories have been advanced by the well-known Swiss, Piaget (1926, 1932, 1958), in his works on the child's language, thought and conception of the world around him. A system basically similar to Piaget's has recently been advanced and described by Sullivan, Grant and Grant (1954). These authors have outlined several levels of integration or development modes of perceiving inter-personal relationships as phases of experience to which all humans are exposed. The authors, after describing the various levels, suggest that not all individuals work their way through each stage but may become fixed at a particular integration level. They give examples of the inter-personal integration of delinquent adults who have failed to make certain discriminations which are held as being essential to character development.

In concluding this particular part of this chapter which aims mainly at describing studies which deal with the *general* background of the delinquency field, it should be mentioned that the hypothetical constructs erected by Freud and his followers until the present time have reigned practically supreme in the field of child development and delinquency. A work of specific relevance is that of Friedlander (1943, 1945, 1946, 1947, 1948, 1949), who has not only summarized the Freudian and neo-Freudian viewpoint on delinquency but has integrated it with her clinical experience and insight.

STUDIES ON PARENT-CHILD RELATIONSHIPS, PARTICULARLY AFFECTION

It is rather surprising to find that despite the fact that experts in the field of child guidance have frequently stressed the importance of home background factors in mental hygiene, there has been a dearth of studies which are systematically and specifically designed to test hypotheses about parent-child relationships. Furthermore, there has been very little effort made to devise psychological tools for the use of workers in child guidance and specifically in children's or juvenile court clinics.

In an attempt to assess the attitude of parents towards their children objectively, it is possible for the research worker to adopt any of the following procedures (Itkin, 1952):

  i. Systematic direct observation of behaviour.
 ii. Systematic case study methods.
iii. Interview methods used to obtain from a child and/or from parents data concerning family relationships as well as factual information.
 iv. Questionnaires.
  v. Self-scoring inventories.
 vi. Projective tests.
vii. Rating scales.

A more detailed approach to attitude testing has been reported on by Oppenheim (1966). Both advantages and disadvantages are attached to each of these methods, but it is possible to use a *combination* of these methods. Earlier it was shown which combination of methods was finally adopted by the writer in carrying out this research, it is here necessary to review the methods used by previous research workers and later to record some of their findings.

It would seem from a review of the literature that one of the finest systematic studies which uses the method of *direct observation of behaviour* is that of Merrill (1946). Two groups of mothers were observed while playing with their children. Merrill then told mothers in the experimental group that their children had not come up to satisfactory standard, while the mothers of the original group were not told this. All mothers were then again observed playing with their children and were rated as to change of attitudes towards their children. It should be mentioned that Buhler (1937) developed a method which makes possible a quantitative analysis of the observations of parents and children. The more recent work of Bandura and Walters, *Social Learning and Personality Development* (1963), exploring among other factors, aggressiveness in children under the impact of television, must not be forgotten, nor that of Himmelweit, Oppenheim, and Vince (1958), and of Berkowitz (1964).

A research worker who used a refinement of the *case-study method* is Fitz-Simons (1935). She employed objective observers in judging parental attitudes from case studies.

Strangely enough, there are rather few *questionnaire-inventory* type of studies. According to Shoben (1949), one of the earliest pioneers in this field was Laws who experimented with this type of technique as early as 1925. Shoben, however, claims that Laws' work did not stand up to present methodological standards of rigor. A questionnaire study which is well known in the U.S.A. is that of Stogdill (1933) who examined differences between mental hygienists and parents in their attitudes about the behaviour of their children. He reports that parents were more alarmed than mental hygienists by such factors as children's misbehaviour, whereas mental hygienists showed more concern about children's deviant behaviour such as withdrawal from other children or from family groups, etc. G. Watson (1933) points out that Stogdill's study is open to severe criticism on methodological grounds.

Shoben's work (1949) is one of the very few existing studies which successfully survives serious criticism. He used the *self-inventory method* and investigated attitudes of 50 mothers of children classed as problem children and 50 mothers of non-problem children. With psychologists acting as judges, his scales were found to be of high reliability. His two major hypotheses are quoted here because they form the centre of all studies of this kind, including that of the present work:

Shoben states:

i. 'It is hypothesized that a given parent behaves toward a given child with sufficient constancy from situation to situation to differentiate himself or herself measurably from other parents. . . .

ii. And it is also hypothesized that the type of characteristic parental behaviour displayed is significantly related to the adjustment of the child.'

He continues by stating: 'If these two ideas are sound it should be possible to construct a measuring device that will differentiate the parents of maladjusted children from the parents of adequately adjusted children.' Shoben proved both his hypotheses to his satisfaction and he makes an observation of considerable importance to the present study. He refers specifically to the attitudes of mothers as well as to the attitudes of fathers, and reports that his study failed to throw enough light on more detailed father-mother relationships. He states: 'Beyond the survey itself, of course, lie a number of problems. . . . Among other questions are such as these: Are specific patterns of parent behaviour associated with specific types of childhood adjustment problems? Do the attitudes of mothers and of fathers differ markedly and what is the relationship between such possible differences and childhood patterns?' It is this latter query raised by Shoben which the writer of this particular thesis was also anxious to subject to detailed investigation.

Another survey which makes use of attitude inventories and which deserves mention is that of Itkin (1952). Itkin studied parent-child relationships by observing a sample of college students and their parents. He concentrated on the validation of such concepts as parental acceptance and rejection and attitudes towards discipline. Validation studies on such concepts have become increasingly common in this field, especially since the work of Champney (1941) has been published. By adopting a Likert scaling procedure (Likert, 1932), Itkin (1952) reports that 'Results . . . appear to support the hypothesis that premarital inter-family factors are significantly related to college students' pre-parental attitudes towards children and suggest the hypothesis that these factors are significantly related to parental attitudes towards children. (The data however . . . concerning aetiology of attitudes towards children . . . suggests that also . . . other factors affect the development of attitudes towards children.' Itkin (1952) draws attention to a factor which seems often overlooked in studies of this kind (and which accordingly was incorporated into the design of this study – namely that 'Caution should be exercised in drawing conclusions as to parental attitudes from reports made by children. Parental behaviour when studied through children's reports should be recognized for what it is – a report of parental behaviour as it is observed by their children, and it cannot be assumed that these reports are perfectly valid indications of underlying parental attitudes. Inaccuracies in children's reports due to emotional and attitudinal factors may introduce a source of error the size of which should be known in evaluating the results of investigations based upon such data.'

Prior to Itkin's study, experimental work in the parent-child relationship field had been reviewed most thoroughly by Symonds (1939). This review includes studies carried out prior to 1939. Stogdill (1936) has surveyed the literature prior to 1936. These studies have of course made use of one or more of the techniques listed on page 141 of this review. It must be remembered that relatively few studies carried out prior to the outbreak of the Second World War can stand up to the strict methodological test that Itkin's study can. Some of those studies which are methodologically sound will be reviewed in greater detail in the following pages. Those many which are not will also be briefly mentioned not so much because of their methodological interest but mainly because of the hypotheses tested which relate to those tested in the study.

Studies which Symonds (1939) has summarized and which are quoted here are Sewell's study of jealousy, Hall's study of children's lies, Zimmermann's work dealing with aggressiveness and timidity in children of rejecting and overprotective mothers; and works on maternal over-protection by Hough, Figge, Lewenberg and Foley. Anderson's (1946) study described the relationships between parents' attitudes and the behaviour of children as did Miles' study (1939) with specific references to the quality of leadership shown by children. Fitz Simon's (1935) study is also of methodological interest and has already been mentioned briefly. By means of his objective scales on case material and reports of independent judges he made interesting contributions towards the understanding of affective relationships between parents and children. He found that (1) the greatest number of withdrawal problems per child occurred in the group containing overprotective mothers and rejecting fathers. (2) That the smallest number of withdrawal problems per child were found in the group in which the mother's attitude was negative towards the child and the father's positive. (3) The greatest number of aggressive behaviour problems were found in a group where both parents were judged as having neglected the child.

Symonds (1939), by working on two major hypotheses, namely, acceptance-rejection and dominance-submissiveness, concluded from the study that: (1) accepted children showed predominantely desirable characteristics and (2) rejected children lack stability, portray attention-getting behaviour, and are inclined to become delinquent, are rebellious and feel persecuted. (3) Children of dominating parents are better socialized, more sensitive, more self-conscious, submissive, orderly, reliable, polite, but more dependent, whereas (4) children of submissive parents are more disorderly, lazy, stubborn, aggressive, but more independent and self-confident. He also found that rejected children tend to come from homes where there is marital disharmony. Regarding the parents and grandparents of these children, he found that dominant parents tend to have been dominated as children by their parents, whereas submissive parents tend to have had parents who were submissive to them.

Kasanin, Knight and Sage (1934) report that maternal overprotection was present in 60% of the 45 cases of schizophrenics which were randomly selected. As mentioned previously in a different connection, Macdonald (1938) found that constructive maternal and paternal attitudes, successful marital adjustment, and the degree of the mothers' insight into their children's problems are important factors in the social adjustment of children. Regarding the relationship between parental personality characteristics and children's behaviour, contradictory findings are reported by Field (1940) and Patterson (1943). Bergum (1940) found that rejected children develop certain characteristics such as independence and early maturity. Martin (1943) in a survey concludes that parental overprotection is more damaging for personality development in children than is parental rejection. As mentioned earlier the question of maternal over-protection has been studied extensively by Levy (1943). Levy's technique is based on the case-study method. He found the following factors operating in the aetiology of maternal over-protection. (1) A long period of anticipation before the birth of a child during which there may have been miscarriage, sterility or abortions. (2) Sexual incompatibility of husband and wife. (3) Affect hunger or insufficient affection during the mother's childhood. (4) Limited social activity of the mother. (5) Assumption of extraordinary responsibilities by the mother during childhood. (6) Thwarted ambitions. (7) Poor health of the child. (8) Ineffectual discipline of the child by the father.

Two series of studies must be briefly mentioned which are complementary to each other, namely, studies of parental attitudes towards children and studies of children's attitudes towards parents. It should be mentioned in passing that the writer has taken account of the fact that studies of this kind are complementary and has, therefore, incorporated them into one single study. The present writer believes that statements of children should be linked with those of parents regarding a particular series of events in order to give more accurate information on child-parent relationships.

Studies on Parental Attitudes towards Children:

Several notable studies on parents' attitudes towards children have been conducted by Read (1945), Coast (1939), Stott (1940, 1940a) and Koch *et al.* (1934), Tennenbaum (1939) and Harris (1948). Read, by using Stogdill's parent-child attitude questionnaire, found that those parents who expressed attitudes favouring freedom towards their children had children who were better adjusted generally. Coast studied attitudes and information of parents of pre-school children concerning praise and corporal punishment. Stott and Koch studied parental attitudes towards discipline. Stott reports no significant differences between the answers about self-reliance given by parents of children in towns and cities and no significant difference between mothers and fathers. Tennenbaum emphasizes the importance of cultural factors in attitudes towards children and concludes that the behaviour of any group of people cannot be adequately understood by reference to individual motivation alone. Harris, in studying change of attitudes, found that present-day attitudes towards children are more liberal than those held 15 years prior to his study. It must be mentioned here that his study (like the present writer's) was not a longitudinal but a cross-sectional one, and therefore Harris could not ultimately assess with certainty any differences that might have occurred in attitudes of parents in the original sample tested in the 15-year period.

Another recent work is that of Kees and Newson (1954). The authors studied the position of a child among his siblings and used a delinquent group and a control group. The authors conclude that the majority of delinquents occupy an intermediate sibling position, and are inclinded to attach themselves to groups. The authors found that a child who is either the only child or the eldest is inclined to be an individualist in the sense that he is the mediator between his parents and his young siblings and deiives satisfaction from this position. They found that the youngest children if threatened can rely on emotional support from their mother. Children who are neither the eldest, not the only child, nor the youngest, lack the satisfaction of being the eldest or trail blazer; nor can they rely on the emotional support from the mother to the extent that the younger child might.

The authors believe that it is for this reason that children who are occupying intermediate position in the sibling family structure are particularly delinquency-prone and inclined to seek satisfaction outside the house by attaching themselves to gangs. They, in fact, feel squeezed out of the home. This situation can be aggravated by poverty where families live in only one or two rooms. Much of this has been more generally confirmed more recently by Schachter (1961).

Studies on Children's Attitudes towards Parents:

Apart from the studies discussed so far concerning parental attitudes towards children, those mentioned in this section concentrate on children's attitudes towards parents. The majority of these studies hypothesize certain affective relationships between a child and his parents, and do not primarily concentrate on such factors as punishment, child ubpringing, etc. Simpson (1935), by utilizing a controlled interview and a projective technique, studied parent preferences of young children. Itkin (1952) summarizes Henry and Emme's study (1939) on college students' attitudes towards their parents. The students were found to have more affection for their mothers than for their fathers; female students had more affection for their parents than had male, and those students who disliked both parents were often maladjusted. An early work of Patrick (1935) also conducted on college students infers that college students view their homes with approval if their parents allow them 'individuality', i.e. parents allowed them to bring their friends home, etc. Zucker (1943) and Hayward (1935) studied parent-child intraparent relationships. Gardner (1947) did research into parental relationships and is one of the very few who studied attitudes towards fathers – a topic of particular relevance to this work. Gardner administered self-scoring questionnaires to schoolboys and girls on a date just prior to Fathers' day (in the U.S.A.) in order to assess their feelings towards their fathers. She reports that one child in six admitted that he had parental preferences. About one child in seven preferred the father to the mother, while one in three preferred the mother. Of the boys who liked the father better than the mother, 64% of them felt that the father understood them better. Of the boys who liked the mother better than the father, 64% of them felt that she understood them better. Regarding punishment, it was found that approximately one-third of punishment was administered by the mother, one-third by the father, and one-third by both parents. Physical punishment was given by the father in 51% of the cases, and by mother in 37% of the cases; and verbal punishment by the father was given in 30% of the cases, and by the mothers in 38% of the cases. Deprivational punishment was given by the father in 19% of the cases, and by the mothers in 25% of the cases. Regarding expression of sibling preferences by parents, 24% of the schoolchildren said that their father preferred another brother or sister to them, and 37% said that their mother preferred another sibling. It was found that parents were inclined to demand most chores from children of the same sex as they were; and also it was found that children did not express special affection for the parent of the opposite sex. Both boys and girls named more ways in which they would like to resemble the parent of the same sex, but rated the parent of the opposite sex higher in character and disposition.

More recent studies on delinquency in particular and children's attitudes towards mothers and fathers in general are that of Oeser Emery and Hammond (1955) and Holman (1953). Holman, who is to a large extent concerned with aetiological questions, finds that surprisingly little attention has been given to the problem of the causes of maladjustment in children, or to comprehensive studies of the various aetiological factors operating in any given type of disorder. Holman's work is somewhat similar to that of Bowlby (1952) in that the concept of 'maternal deprivation' is studied. Also studied is the role and relationship of the father. She infers that while Bowlby's findings are basically sound, the concept of deprivation may do social harm because it is essentially a negative one. Her findings with regard to such factors as aggression, broken homes, etc., agree in general with the findings of research workers which have been discussed so far. She concludes that while it was not possible to establish the relative importance of different aetiological factors in aggressive behaviour, the following factors are important to adequate adjustment: (1) the type of mother-father relationship, (2) the parental attitudes towards the child, (3) permanent early separation from one or both parents.

In this brief review of the literature it will now be necessary to discuss relatively rather more recent studies which stand out not only for their sound methodological approach but also for the hypotheses which are tested. One such study is that of Radke (1946) who studied the relation of parental authority to children's behaviour and attitudes. A mixture of techniques was used (interview, rating scales, etc.). Factors such as discipline, parental affect, were investigated. Radke concludes that the 'study of relationships between home atmosphere and teachers' ratings of children's behaviour gives evidence that the child carries over in his own behaviour to other children the behaviour of his parents. Thus, it appears that in order to obtain desired behaviour from the child, the parent must manifest such behaviour himself.'

A study which deserves particular mention because of its special findings and systematic design is that of Champney (1941) who devised a series of parent behaviour attitude scales of considerable sensitivity. The work was carried out by him at the Samuel Fels Research Institute, Ohio, and the scales are consequently known as the Fels Scales, work which has later been carried on by Kagan and Moss (1962), and Kagan, Mussen, and Conger (1964, 1970). Champney mapped out a series of areas in the field of family relationships such as affect, democracy, child centredness in the home, readiness of enforcement of rules, etc. Each of these areas are carefully defined and bipolar points are fixed at the extremes of the scales. Thus the scale is designed in such a way that the possibility of intuitive judgement is reduced to a minimum. The scales and the method of application are described by Baldwin, Kalhorn and Breese (1945). The underlying hypotheses which Champney ultimately proved (and which seems a fitting conclusion to the review of the literature) were stated by him as follows:

'A given parent behaves towards a given child in certain ways which (*a*) tend to be consistent from situation to situation, and (*b*) tend to differentiate him from other parents. Such consistently repeated situations are for the child learning situations in which social habits are formed, developed and generalized into the habit systems which at length constitute his adult personality.'

Further Studies on Affective Relationships between Parents and Children (including those on separations)

In the decade since the original version of this book came out, several additional important researches have been published. These tend to confirm Bowlby's original thesis that in certain circumstances the so-called 'maternal deprivation' factor can be harmful and give rise to delinquent behaviour. However, they also tend increasingly to confirm the author's general hypothesis, namely that paternal relationships are also of immense importance here, and that genetic and cross-cultural and inter-personal relationships each have a subtle part to play (W.H.O. Monograph No. 14, 1962 *Deprivation of Maternal Care: a reassessment of its effects*, Ainsworth, Andry, et al.; also *Maternal Care and Deprivation*, Bowlby, Ainsworth, Andry, et al., 1967). Further, such works show that complex relationships between factors cannot best be demonstrated by simple observation, but require studies with adequate controls, the use of simple correlation orchai square techniques, but preferably require more advanced psychometric techniques, including those based on factor-analysis, as shown among others by R. G. Andry (1963), G. Trasler (1962), C. Banks and P. Broadhurst (1965).

Here Bowlby's own more recent works in this field should also be mentioned (Bowlby, Vols. I and II, 1969), where among other factors following the work of Harlow (1962) he points out that there is a similarity between the behaviour of infants and certain innate clinging responses of monkeys who were separated from their mothers and were undergoing significant 'mourning' processes, with the resultant danger, in extreme cases, of becoming 'affectionless' characters. Harlow's own works (1962 op. cit.) in this field have become classics showing that young monkeys who were separated from their mothers when given the choice between finding solace by either going to an artificial 'wire mother', one with a built in food-giving device, or to another artificial and padded mother without the food-giving device, tended to seek comfort rather than food from the padded 'substitute mother'. This tends to show the supremacy of the comforting over the food-seeking drive within certain experimental limitations, and probably shows the importance of personality differences as has been indirectly pointed out by the author (1963), and by Eysenck (1970).

Also, mention must be made here of the impressive researches edited by Foss (1961, 1963, 1969), partly in conjunction with Bowlby giving details, among others, of the work of Gewirtz in relation to infantile smiling responses and supporting interesting trends in this field, recorded by the Hoffmanns (1964 and 1966).

The Gluecks, with their impressive industriousness, have not stood idle during the last decade and have not only followed up some of their original predictive studies (1950), but among several of their works have been pioneering the work of the role played by physique and delinquency (1956), and on typology (1970). A useful general review covering forty-five references on the topic of separation was recently completed by Munro (1969).

Particular aspects, including father–child relationships, following the writer's work in 1960, have been reported on by, among others, B. Frost (1962), and by R. Andry in relation to team work in Grygier, Spencer and Jones (1965), and more specifically in the psycho-analytical field by Winnicott (1965), Hyatt Williams (in H. Klare and D. Haxby (1967)), and R. D. Laing (1966) and 1960 in his *Divided Self*.

Apart from these general works, there are some of special interest which deal with child–parent separation problems. For instance Naess (*British Journal of Delinquency*, 1959–60), carried out research into the relevant question of why the deprivation–separation factor affects some but not all siblings in the same family. He, by matching delinquents and non-delinquent siblings, found that the deprivation factor in relation to delinquency *per se* was not significantly correlated. This has been indirectly confirmed by M. Power (1966) and J. W. B. Douglas et al. (1968) and Douglas (1964), and measured with a special instrument assessing family interaction, and A. Little (*British Journal of Criminology*, 1965). Also Burton and Whiting (1961) in a cross-cultural study found that children deprived of fathers, especially boys, tend to suffer from sex-role identification problems. Lynn and Sawrey (1959), in studying the effect of irregular absence of fathers on children of Norwegian sailors found that deprived boys tended to be more immature than their non-deprived peers, that father-deprived girls tended to become excessively mother-dependant, and that these children become generally more disturbed.

The whole topic was also taken up more directly by Leslie Wilkins under the heading of 'Delinquent Generation' Wilkins (1964). His work links up with Andry's general hypothesis about the 'paternal deprivation' effect on children by specifically examining whether children at around five years of age who have suffered 'paternal deprivation' (especially while fathers were abroad on war service), are likely to show a greater than usual propensity of delinquent behaviour in later life. A retrospective study by examining adolescent delinquents tended to confirm this hypothesis. This was also later confirmed by other cross-cultural studies, including one from New Zealand and reported on in several issues of the *British Journal of Criminology*, though followed through more recently by a rejoinder from G. N. G. Rose, 'The Artificial Delinquent Generation' (1968).

Further Studies Related to possible Constitutional Factors in Delinquency

Following the trend set by Lombroso (op. cit.) (who with his 'atavism' theory tended to see much of the origin of criminality in terms of inborn constitutional factors), the majority of criminologists (largely under the influence of Freud's psychoanalytical environmental and sociological thinking) have tended until recently to neglect almost entirely the role of genetics in this field.

Eysenck, *Crime and Personality* (1970) was one of the first during the last decade to help reverse this trend to some extent, not only by giving results of his own researches and those of his followers (e.g. Franks, 1970), but also by drawing readers' attention to such well-known researches by Shields (1962), Lange (1970) and others.

These findings dovetailed to some extent with the work of, among others, Mary Woodward (1955), who helped to convince those who had not already been familiar with similar American and Australian studies of a decade earlier, that the majority of delinquents *per se* were not necessarily of low inborn intelligence. That intelligence among disturbed delinquents can fluctuate depending on educational opportunity was demonstrated more recently by, among others, J. W. B. Douglas (1968) and by Donald West (*Present Conduct and Future Delinquency*, 1969) and T. Veness (1962).

The role of minimal brain damage through E.E.G. investigations has received attention in this field largely through the findings of Russell Davies (1966). This could help to exonerate, at least to a certain extent, some parents as faulty educators of potential delinquents.

The Gluecks (*Physique and Delinquency*, 1956) have also pointed out the likely genetic relationship with certain types of delinquents between their mesomorphic body build and their delinquent behaviour, as did the writer in connection with the extroverted and extrapunitive type of behaviour displayed among certain recidivists (R. G. Andry, *The Short-term Prisoner*, 1963).

Even more recently, some researchers (see Sarbin and Miller in *Issues in Criminology*, Summer 1970) have reported chromosome abnormalities among some, usually tall and often mentally retarded, recidivists who often seem to have one or even more additional masculine 'Y'-type chromosomes in their structure. Alternatively, they can, on occasion, also show abnormalities in the feminine determining 'X' factors by double or multiple 'X' factors having occurred among male delinquents.

Endocrinological and biochemical investigations have scarcely begun in the field of criminology but it might be speculated that similar to those of the geneticists, these may come to the fore during the next decade.

Further Studies Related to Parent-child Training Problems

Apart from genetic and affective relationship variables, probably the single most important other variable is that of parent–child training. It has been hypothesized over decades that if parents during the first formative years of their children's lives train, educate and bring them up equitably and morally, then the likelihood of such children not turning into delinquents is considerable. Thus, there are many studies which have tended to show that if 'training' has been poor on the part of the parent (or substitutes, including grandparents), then there is a greater-than-chance likelihood of delinquent behaviour being manifested by such children. Alternatively, there may be genetic in-born or 'imprinting' predisposition periods when child-training may be more effective at early critical times than later in a child's development. This area of study can thus be divided technically into several subsections: (a) wrong training which can effect the faulty conscious ego or super ego development and lead to character malformation (following the works of Freud, see C. S. Hall, 1956), and absence of remorse (Kohlberg, 1966); or, (b) aggression and violence (Wolfgang and Ferracuti, 1967, and McClintock, 1963) which includes the classical study of the McCords (1959). McCord and McCord for instance showed, with their six-fold table, that violence tends to breed violence and that above all, parents lacking in training consistency are in danger of indirectly encouraging delinquency. Similarly, the Hoffmans (1964 and 1966) distinguish between three different types among delinquents following faulty training: an external one (who judges merely in terms of punishment), a conventional one (as an upholder of rules) and a humanist one (who judges in terms of consequences to the interest and feelings of others). This may or may not be considered an improvement on Hewitt and Jenkins (1947) earlier triple factor hypothesis which talked of an unsocialized aggressive type, a socialised, and an over-inhibited one, all lately critically researched into by Joy Mott (1967 in Klare and Haxby).

This is in contrast to Hartshorn and May's (1930) earlier single factor theory of 'honesty–dishonesty' which subsequent research failed to support. Apart from Trasler (1962), work in the factor–analytical field on this topic has also been carried out by Schaefer (1959). His bi-polar factor theory of child rearing techniques distinguishes between the love–hostility variable, and that of control-autonomy, suggesting that over-demonstrative parents are often scoring high on the love but low on the control variables. This work has been extended by Becker, et al. (1962) who further subdivided the second 'control-autonomy' variable into a third factor of restrictiveness versus persuasiveness and anxious versus calm-and-detached. He suggested that certain delinquents had parents who had brought them up at the extremes of these variables; that is, were either too restrictive or too permissive, or too anxious or too calm in their up-bringing techniques.

Following Piaget's (1932) original work (see also Ruth Beard, 1969) which hypothesized 'stages' over periods of years in the development of moral judgement of a child (accompanied in delinquents by the possibility of parents' inability to recognise the critical moments in the development of these stages) it must be recalled that Piaget suggested that the seven-years-old stage is crucial in the moral development of a young child. Further work by Kohlberg (in E. E. Maccoby (Ed.) 1966) confirms Piaget's findings but suggests the existence of three moral developmental stages: an infantile pre-moral one, followed by a conventional role conforming one which may lead to one of 'self-acceptance'. This work was extended further by Grim, Kohlberg and Whyte (1964, see Hoffman, 1964) leading to a five-stage framework, not dissimilar to that of Peck and of Havighurst's (1960) five developmental stages (ranging from the amoral via the expedient, the conforming, the irrational to the altruistic-rationless stage). The similarity here again is obvious between these findings and those of Sullivan, Grant and Grant (1954) and of the author (Andry op. cit., 1963). Also of interest in the training field is the work of R. W. Shields (1962) and of R. G. Andry (1968) in relation to legal aspects in this field. Thus practically everything tends to point to the need for further research to try and match those who are somewhat arrested at a more primitive 'moral developmental' stage with those experts of an appropriately higher moral developmental stage who may be capable of training delinquents to achieve subsequent higher developmental stages.

Further Studies Related to Child-parent and General Communication Problems and the Role of Group Dynamics

There is an ever increasing need to bridge the gap between the criminological, sociological and the psychological literatures. It is thus beyond the scope of this book to give a detailed review of recent advances in these fields other than to point out a few major trend-setting directions.

In the field of sociology, a number of interesting trends have emerged (see Barbara Wootton, 1959) such as those set by Matza (1969) who believes less than his colleagues in the existence of a delinquency sub-culture, by Kitsuse (1963) who examines the arbitrary way of 'labelling' value orientated techniques of delinquents by society (A. Cicourel, 1968), by A. Cohen (1966) and by Bernstein (1965) who has drawn attention to the differences in the usage of linguistic codes among various socio-economic classes in their communication efforts between parents, children, teachers and other educators.

In psychology a great deal of research has taken place which deals with relevant topics such as (a) attitude formation (see Krech, Crutchfield and Ballachey (1962), Roger Brown (1965), Secord and Bachman (1964), or Lindzsey and Aronson (1969)) and (b) role playing techniques both on the part of parents, children, and the expected role behaviour by society with resultant conflict possibilities as summarised by Biddle and Thomas (1966), and (c) motivation, especially the achievement motivation (McClelland, 1961) (d) communication (see Watzlawick et al., 1968) and (e) research (see H. C. Quay, 1965), B. A. Maher (1964–67), I. A. Berg and B. M. Bass (1961), and see J. G. Howells (1965), and (f) social class and delinquency (Lynn McDonald (1969), (g) legal implications (Andry, 1965), also see Carmichael's *Child Psychology* (1963). Whether acknowledged or not, a great deal of these works go back to theoretical foundations either of the behaviourists, on in particular, the neo-Gestaltist or field theorists, especially of Kurt Lewin (1936, 1948). Related to this is also the position advanced by psychoanalytically orientated workers, such as Slavson (1965), Bion (1965), Foulkes (1965), who point out that delinquent, like any other behaviour, can best be studied (and cured, depending on circumstances) through the group, be it that of the total family (Andry, *GAIPAC Journal* (1969, 1970)) or in therapeutic probation-type groups (Klare, Andry et al., in *Howard Journal*, article in preparation).

To be effective, it is once again obvious that careful assessment and 'classification' of delinquents is required before allocating them to different types of treatment regimes (Andry, *The Short-term Prisoner*), be it individual, group or other forms of therapies (including behaviour therapy as described by Beech, 1969). Thus, it is here predicted (following the experience of the previous decade) that the next decade is less likely to produce radically new ideas in this field but will show instead a greater preoccupation with more carefully controlled experiments.

2 : BIBLIOGRAPHY

AICHHORN, A. 1936. *Wayward Youth*. London: Putnam

ALEXANDER, F. and STAUB, H. 1931. *The Criminal, the Judge, and the Public: A Psychological Analysis*. New York: Macmillan

ANDERSON, J. E. 1946. 'Parents' attitudes on Child Behaviour: A report of three studies.' *Child Devel.*, **17**, 91–97

ANDRIOLA, J. 1946. 'The Truancy Syndrome.' *Amer. J. Ortho. Psychiat.*, **16**, 174

ANDRY, R. G. 1957. 'Faulty Paternal and Maternal Child Relationships, Affection and Delinquency.' *The Brit. J. of Del.* **5**, No. 1

ANDRY, R. G. 1963. *The Short Term Prisoner*. London: Stevens

ANDRY, R. G. 'Legal Implications in Parent-Child Relationships'. See Emmanuel Miller (Ed.). 1968. *Foundations in Child Psychiatry*. Oxford: Pergamon

ANDRY, R. G. 1969–70. 'Family relationships, learning and therapy.' *GAIPAC Journal*

ANDRY, R. G. *Forensic Psychology*. In preparation

ARGYLE, M. 1964. *Psychology and Social Problems*. London: Methuen

ARGYLE, M. 1967. *Psychology of Interpersonal Behaviour*. Penguin

ARGYLE, M. 1969. *Social Interaction*. London: Methuen

BALDWIN, A. L., KALHORN, J. and REESE, F. H. 1945. 'Patterns of Parent Behaviour.' *Psychol. Monogr.*, **58**, 1–75

BANDURA, A. and WALTERS, R. H. 1963. *Social Learning and Personality Development*. New York: Holt, Rinehart & Winston

BANNISTER, H. and RAVDEN, M. 1944. 'The Problem Child and his Environment.' *Brit. J. Psychol. (Gen. Section)*, **34**, Part II

BEARD, R. 1969. *An Outline of Piaget's Development Psychology*. London: Routledge & Kegan Paul

BECKER, W. C. et al. 1962. 'Relations of factors derived from parent-interview ratings to behaviour problems of five-year olds'. *Child Develop.*, **33**, 509–535

BEECH, H. R. 1969. *Changing Man's Behaviour*. Harmondsworth, Middx.: Penguin

BENDER, L. and SCHILDER, P. 1937. 'Suicidal preoccupations and attempts in children.' *Amer. J. Ortho. Psychiat.*, **7**, 225

BENNETT, I. V. P. 1951. *A Comparative Study of Delinquent and Neurotic Children*. Unpub. Ph.D. thesis. Univ. of London

BENNETT, I. V. P. 1960. *Delinquent & Neurotic Children: a comparative study*. London: Tavistock Pubns

BERG, I. A. and BASS, B. M. 1961. *Conformity and Deviation*. New York: Harper

BERGUM, M. 1940. 'Constructive values associated with rejection.' *Amer. J. Ortho. Psychiat.*, **10**, 312–327

BERKOWITZ, L. 1962. *Aggression: a social psychological analysis.* New York: McGraw-Hill

BERKOWITZ, L. 1964. *The Development of Motives and Values in the Child.* New York, London: Basic Books

BERNSTEIN, B: 1965. 'A Socio-Linguistic Approach to Social Learning.' *Social Science Survey*

BIDDLE, B. J. and THOMAS, E. J. 1966. *Role Theory.* New York: Wiley

BION, W. R. 1965. *Transformation.* London: Heinemann

BOWLBY, J. 1944. *Intern. J. Psychoanal.*, **25**, 19

BOWLBY, J. 1946. *Forty-four Juvenile Thieves; Their Characters and Home Life.* London: Ballière, Tindall & Cox

BOWLBY, J. 1952. *Maternal Care and Mental Health.* World Health Organ. Monogr. Geneva

BOWLBY, J., ANDRY, R. G. and AINSWORTH, M. 1962. *Deprivation of Maternal Care: A reassessment of its effects.* W.H.O. Public Health Papers, No. 14

BOWLBY, J. 1965. *Child Care and the Growth of Love.* Harmondsworth, Middx.: Penguin

BOWLBY, J., AINSWORTH, M., ANDRY, R. G. et al. 1967. *Maternal Care and Deprivation.* New York: Schocken Books

BOWLBY, J. 1969. *Attachment and Loss* (2 Vols). London: Hogarth Press

BROWN, R. 1965. *Social Psychology.* New York: Free Press of Glencoe. London: Collier-Macmillan

BUHLER, C. 1937. *The Child and his family.* New York: Harper

BURLINGHAM, D. and FREUD, A. 1942. *Young Children in Wartime in a Residential War Nursery.* London: Allen & Unwin

BURLINGHAM, D. and FREUD, A. 1943. *Infants without Families.* London: Allen & Unwin

BURT, C. 1925. *The Psychology of the Young Criminal.* Howard League Pamphlets, No. 4

BURT, C. 1925. *The Young Delinquent.* London, 4th edition, 1944. Univ. of London Press

BURTON, R. V. and WHITING, J. W. M. 1961. 'The Absent Father and Cross-Sex Identity'. *Merrill-Palmer Quart.* **7**, 85–95

CARMICHAEL, L. 1963. *Manual of Child Psychology.* New York: Wiley

CARR-SAUNDERS, A. M., MANNHEIM, H. and RHODES, E. C. 1942. *Young Offenders: An Enquiry into Juvenile Delinquency.* Cambridge Univ. Press

CAWSON, A., COOPER, E., COOPER, J. E. and DOUGLAS, J. W. B. 1968. 'Family Interaction and the Activities of Young Children'. *5 Child/ Psychiat.* 157–171

CHAMPNEY, H. 1941. 'The Measurement of Parent Behaviour.' *Child Develop.*, **12**, 131–166

CHAMPNEY, H. 1941. 'The Variables of Parent Behaviour.' *J. Abnorm. Soc. Psych.*, **36**, 525–542

CHILDERS, A. T. and HAMIL, B. M. 1932. 'Emotional Problems in Children as related to the duration of breast feeding in infancy.' *Amer. J. Ortho. Psychiat.*, **2**, 134

CICOUREL, A. 1968. *The Social Organization of Juvenile Justice.* New York: Wiley

CLAYBORNE, R. B. 1954. *Study of Parent Attitudes in Juvenile Delinquency.* Abstract of Ph.D. thesis: School of Education, New York University

COAST, L. C. 1939. 'A Study of the knowledge and attitudes of parents of pre-school children.' *Stud. Child Welf.*, **17**, 175–191

COHEN, A. 1966. *Deviance and Control.* New York: Prentice-Hall

CLOWARD, R. A. and OHLIN, L. E. 1961. *Delinquency and Opportunity.* London: Routledge & Kegan Paul

CLYNE, M. B. 1966. *Absent.* London: Tavistock Publications

DAVIES, R. 1966. Introduction to Psychopathology. London: Oxford University Press

DOUGLAS, J. W. B. 1964. *The Home and the School.* London: MacGibbon & Kee

DOUGLAS, J. W. B. et al. 1968. *All Our Future.* P. Davies

DOWNES, D. M. 1966. *The Delinquent Situation.* London: Routledge & Kegan Paul

EYSENCK, H. J. 1970. *Crime and Personality.* London: Paladin

FENICHEL, OTTO. 1934. *Outline of Clinical Psycho-analysis.* New York: Norton & Co.

FIELD, M. 1940. 'Maternal attitudes found in twenty-five cases of children with primary behaviour disorders. *Amer. J. Ortho. Psychiat.*, **10**, 293–312

FIGGE, M. see Symonds

FITZ-SIMONS M. J. 1935. *Some Parent-child Relationships as shown in Clinical. Case Studies.* New York: Teach. Coll. Columbia Univ.

FOSS, B. 1961, 1963 and 1969. *Determinants of Infant Behaviour.* London: Methuen

FOULKES, S. H. and ANTHONY, E. G. 1965. *Group Psychotherapy.* Harmondsworth, Middx.: Penguin

FRANKS, C. see H. J. EYSENCK. *Crime and Personality.* London: Paladin

FREUD, S. 1917. 'Mourning and Melancholia.' *Collected Papers*, **4**, 152. London: Hogarth Press

FREUD, S. 1949. *An Outline of Psychoanalysis.* London: Hogarth Press

FRIEDLANDER, K. 1943. *Delinquency Research. The new era*

FRIEDLANDER, K. 1945. 'Formation of the anti-social character.' *Psychoanal Study of Child*, **1**, 189

FRIEDLANDER, K. 1946. 'Psychoanalytic orientation in child guidance work in Great Britain.' *Psychoanal Study of Child.*, **2**, 343

FRIEDLANDER, K. 1947. *The Psychoanalytical Approach to Juvenile Delinquency.* London: Routledge

FRIEDLANDER, K. 1948. 'The significance of the home in emotional growth.' *The New Era.*, **29**, No. 3

FRIEDLANDER, K. 1949. *Latent Delinquency and ego development. Searchlights on Delinquency: New Psychoanalytic Studies.* Ed. K. R. Rissler. London: Imago

FROMMER, E. 1969. *Voyage through Childhood into the Adult World: a Description of Child Development*. Oxford: Pergamon

FROMMER, E. 1969. *Depressive Illness in Childhood: Recent Developments in Affective Disorders*. Ed. Kopin and Walk. Pergamon. Royal Medico-Pshchological Soc. Special publication of the *Brit. J. Psychiatry*. 1968

FROST, B. 1962. 'The Pattern of WISC Scores in a Group of Juvenile Sociopaths'. *J. Clin. Psychol.* **18**, 354–355

GARDNER, L. P. 1947. 'The analysis of children's attitudes towards fathers.' *J. Genet. Psychol.*, **70**, 3–28

GESELL, A. et al. 1940. *The First Five Years of Life*. London: Methuen

GEWIRTZ, J. L. 'The Course of Smiling by Groups of Israeli Infants in the First Eighteen Months of Life'. In *Studies in Psychology, Scripta Hierosolymitana*, **14**, Jerusalem: Hebrew University Press

GLOVER, E. 1933. *War, Sadism, and Pacifism*. London: Allen & Unwin

GLOVER, E. 1949. *Psycho-Analysis*. London: Staples Press

GLUECK, S. and E. 1950. *Unravelling Juvenile Delinquency*. New York: the Commonwealth Fund

GLUECK, S. and E. 1956. *Physique and Delinquency*. New York: Harper

GLUECK, S. and E. 1970. *Toward a Typology of Juvenile Offenders*. New York: Grune and Stratton

GOLDBERG, E. M. 1958. *Family Influences and Psychosomatic Illness*. London: Tavistock Publications

GOLDMAN, F. 1948. 'Breast feeding and character formation.' *J. Person.*, **17**, No. 1

GOODMAN, S. E. and MICHAELS, J. E. 1934. 'Incidence intercorrelations of enuresis and other neuro-pathic traits in so-called normal children.' *Amer. J. Ortho. Psychiat.*, **4**, 79

GRIM, P., KOHLBERG, L. and WHYTE, S. 1964. *Some Relationships between Conscience and Attentional Processes*. Unpublished paper. (See Hoffman Vol. I. 1964)

GRYGIER, T. 1955. 'Leisure pursuits of juvenile delinquents: a study in methodology.' *Brit. J. Del.*, **5**, No. 3

GRYGIER, J., SPENCER, J. C. and JONES, K. 1965. *Criminology in Transition*. London: Tavistock Publications

HALL, C. S. 1956. *A Primer of Freudian Psychology*. London: Allen and Unwin

HALL, D. see Symonds

HALL, J. and JONES, D. C. 1950. 'Social grading of occupations.' *Brit. J. Soc.*, **1**, 31–55

HALL-WILLIAMS, J. E. 1970. *The English Penal System in Transition*. London: Butterworth

HARLOW, H. F. 1962. 'Social Deprivation in Monkeys'. Reprinted from *Scientific American*

HARRIS, D. B. 1948. 'Social change in the beliefs of adults concerning parent-child relationships.' *American Psychologist*, **3**, 264

HARTSTHORN, H. and MAY, M. A. 1928–30. *Studies in the Nature of Character:* Vol. I: Studies in Deceit; Vol. II: Studies in Self-Control;

Vol. III: Studies in the Organization of Character. New York: Macmillan

HAYWARD, R. S. 1935. 'Child's report of psychological factors in the family.' *Arch. Psych.* **189**, 1–75

HEALY, W. 1915. *The Individual Delinquent.* London: Heinemann

HEALY, W. and BRONNER, A. F. 1925. *Delinquents and Criminals: Their Making and Unmaking.* New York: Macmillan

HEALY, W. and BRONNER, A. F. 1936. *New Light on Delinquency, and its Treatment.* New Haven: Yale Univ. Press

HENRY, L. K. and EMME, E. E. 1939. 'The home adjustment inventory: an attitude scale for personnel procedures.' *Psychol. Bul.*, **36**, 630

HEWITT, L. E. and JENKINS, R. L. 1947. *Fundamental Patterns of Maladjustment: the dynamics of their origin.* Illinois: Springfield

HIMMELWEIT, H. and SUMMERFIELD, A. 1951. 'Student selection: an experimental investigation III.' *Brit. J. Soc.*, **8, 6**, 340

HIMMELWEIT, H. T., OPPENHEIM, A. N. and VINCE, P. 1958. *Television and the Child.* New York: Oxford University Press

HOFFMAN, M. L. and L. W. Vol. I (1964) and Vol. II (1966). *Review of Child Development Research.* New York: Russell Sage Foundation

HOLMAN, P. 1953. 'Some factors in the aetiology of maladjustment in children. *J. Ment. Sci.*, **99**, 654–688

HOUGH, G. see Symonds

HOWELLS, J. G. 1965. *Modern Perspectives in Child Psychiatry.* Edinburgh: Oliver & Boyd

A. HYATT WILLIAMS. see H. KLARE & D. HAXBY. *Frontiers of Criminology.* Oxford: Pergamon. 1970

ITKINS, N. W. 'Some relationships between intra-family attitudes, and pre-parental attitudes toward children.' *J. Genet. Psychol.*, **80**, 221–252

JONES, H. 1962. *Crime and the Penal System.* University Tutorial Press

KAGAN, J. and MOSS, H. A. 1962. *Birth to Maturity: the Fels study of psychological development.* New York: Wiley

KAGAN, J., MUSSEN, P. H. and CONGER, J. J. 1964. *Child Development and Personality.* New York: Harper & Row

KAGAN, J., MUSSEN, P. H. and CONGER, J. J. 1970. *Readings in Child Development and Personality.* New York: Harper & Row

KARPMAN, B. 1948. 'Conscience in the psychopath: another version.' *Amer. J. Ortho. Psychiat.*, **18**, 455

KARPMAN, B. 1948. 'Milestones in the advancement of knowledge of the psychopathology of delinquency and crime.' (in) *Orthopsychiatry 1923–1948. Retrospect and Prospect.* pp. 100. Ed. Lowrey, L. G. & Sloane, V

KASININ, J., KNIGHT, E. and SAGE, P. 1934. 'The parent-child relationship in schizophrenia. I Overprotection-rejection.' *J. Nerv. Ment. Dis.*, **79**, 249–263. Quoted by Itkin

KITSUSE, J. I. and CICOUREL, A. 1963. *The Educational Decision Makers.* Indianapolis: Bobbs-Merrill

KLARE, H. and HAXBY, D. 1967. *Frontiers of Criminology*. Oxford: Pergamon

KLARE, H., ANDRY, R. G. et al. *The Howard Journal*. Article in preparation. 1971

KLEIN, M. 1932. *The Psychoanalysis of Children*. London: Hogarth

KOCH, H. L., DENTLER, M., DYSART, B. and STRAIT, H. 'A scale for measuring attitude, towards the question of children's freedom.' *Child Develop.*, **5**, 252–266.

KOHLBERG, L. 1966. 'Sex Differences in Morality'. *The Development of Sex Differences*. E. E. Maccoby (Ed). Stanford, California: Stanford University Press

KRECH, D., CRUTCHFIELD, R. and BALLACHEY, E. L. 1962. *Individual in Society*. New York: McGraw-Hill

LAING, R. D. 1960. *The Divided Self: a study of sanity and madness*. London: Tavistock Publications

LAING, R. D. 1966. *Interpersonal Perception*. London: Tavistock Publications

LANGE, O. 1970. *Theory of Reproduction and Accumulation*. Oxford: Pergamon

LAWTON, D. 1969. *Social Class, Language and Education*. London: Routledge & Kegan Paul

LEES, J. P. and NEWSON, L. J. 1954. 'Family and sibship position and some aspects of juvenile delinquents.' *Brit. J. Delin.*, **5**, No. 1

LEVY, D. M. 1937. 'Primary Affect Hunger.' *Amer. J. Psychiat.*, **94**, 643–652

LEVY, D. M. 1943. *Maternal Overprotection.* New York: Columbia Univ. Press

LEWENBERG, S. and FOLEY, K. see Symonds

LEWIN, K. et al. 1939. 'Patterns of aggressive behaviour in experimentally created social climates.' *J. Soc. Psychol*, **10**, 271–299

LEWIN, K. 1936. *Principles of Topological Psychology*. New York: McGraw-Hill.

LEWIN, K. 1948. *Resolving Social Conflicts:* selected papers on group dynamics. New York: Harper

LIKERT, A. 1932. 'A technique for the measurement of attitudes.' *Arch. Psych.* **22**, 5–55

LINDNER, R. M. 1971. *Rebel Without a Cause*. Harmondsworth: Penguin

LINDZEY, G. and ARONSON, E. 1969. *The Handbook of Social Psychology*. In 5 vols. Reading, Mass: Addison-Wesley

LIPPMAN, H. S. 1937. 'The neurotic delinquent.' *Amer. J. Ortho. Psychiat.*, **7**, 114

LIPPMAN, H. S. 1945. 'Treatment of Aggression: Psychoanalytical.' *Amer. J. Ortho. Psychiat.*, **13**, 415

LITTLE, A. 'The Increase in Crime 1952–62: An Empirical Analysis of Adolescent Offenders'. *Brit. J. Crim.* (1965) **5**, 77–82

LOMBROSO, C. 1918. '*Crime, its Causes and Remedies*.' Eng. trans. Henry P. Horton, Boston

LOWRY, L. G. 1936. 'The family as a builder of personality.' *Amer. J. Ortho. Psychiat.*, **6**, 117

LYNN, D. B. and SAWREY, W. L. 1959. 'The Effects of Father Absence on Norwegian Boys and Girls'. *J. Abnorm. Soc. Pyschol.* **59**, 258–62

MACDONALD, M. W. 1938. 'Criminally aggressive behaviour in passive effeminate boys.' *Amer. J. Ortho. Pyschiat.*, **8**, 70

MAHER, B. A. 1964–7. *Progress in Experimental Personality Research.* Vols. 1–4. New York: Academic Press

MAKARENKO, A. 1936. *The Road to Life.* London: Lindsay Drummond.

MANNHEIM, H. 1948. *Juvenile Delinquency In An English Middletown.* London: Kegan Paul

MANNHEIM, H. 1949. 'The limits of present knowledge' (in) *Why Delinquency?* The Case for Operational Research. Report of a Conference on the Scientific Study of Juvenile Delinquency. p. 10. L.A.M.N., London

MANNHEIM, H. and WILKINS, L. T. 1955. *Prediction Methods In Relation To Borstal Training.* London: H.M.S.O.

MANNHEIM, H. 1965. *Comparative Criminology.* London: Routledge & Kegan Paul

MARTIN, A. R. 1943. 'A study of parental attitudes and their influence upon personality development.' Educ. Boston, **63**, 596–608. Quoted by Itkin

MATZA, D. 1969. *Becoming Deviant.* Englewood Cliffs: Prentice-Hall

MAYS, J. B. 1955. *Growing Up In A City.* Univ. of Liverpool

MAYS, J. B. 1971. *Juvenile Delinquency: The Family and the Social Group.* London: Longmans

MCCLELLAND, D. C. 1961. *The Achieving Society.* London: Van Nostrand

MCCLINTOCK, F. H. 1963. 'Crimes of Violence'. Camb. Inst. of Crim.

MCCORD, W. and J. 1959. *Origins of Crime: a new evaluation of the Cambridge-Somerville Youth Study.* New York: Columbia U.P.

MCDONALD, L. 1969. *Social Class and Delinquency.* London: Faber & Faber

MCDOUGALL, W. 1932. The Energies of Men: A Study of the Fundamentals of Dynamic Psychology. London: Methuen

MCNEMAR, A. 1949. *Psychological Statistics.* New York: John Wiley & Sons. London: Chapman & Hall

MENNINGER, K. A. 1930. *The Human Mind.* New York: Knopf

MERRILL, B. 1946. 'A measurement of mother-child interaction.' *J. Abnorm. Soc. Psych.*, **41**, 37–49

MICHAELS, J. C. 1938. 'The incidence of enuresis and age of cessation in 100 delinquents and 100 sibling controls.' *Amer. J. Ortho. Psychiat.*, **8**, 46

MILES, O. see Symonds

MORENO, J. *Sociometry and the Science of Man.* New York: Beacon House

MORRIS, N. and HAWKER, G. 1969. *The Honest Politicians Guide to Crime Control.* University of Chicago Press

MORRIS, T. P. 1958. *The Criminal Area—A Study in Social Ecology.* London: Routledge

MOTT, J. see H. KLARE and D. HAXBY. 1967. *Frontiers of Criminology.* Oxford: Pergamon

MOWRER, O. H. and MOWRER, W. M. 1938. 'Enuresis: a method for its study and treatment.' *Amer. J. Ortho. Psychiat.*, **8,** 436

MUNRO, 1969. *General Psychiatry.* **20,** 598

NAESS, S. 1959–60. 'Mother-Child Separation and Delinquency'. *Brit. J. Delin.* Vol. **10,** p. 22

NEWELL, H. W. 1934. 'The psychodynamics of maternal rejection.' *Amer. J. Ortho. Psychiat.*, **4,** 387

NEWELL, H. W. 1936. 'A further study of maternal rejection.' *Amer. J. Ortho. Psychiat.*, **6,** 576

OESER, O. H., EMERY, F. and HAMMOND, S. 1955. *Social Structure and Personality.* 2 Vols. London: Kegan Paul

OPPENHEIM, A. N. 1966. *Questionnaire Design and Attitude Measurement.* London: Heinemann

PATRICK, J. G. 1935. 'The role of intimate groups in the personality development of selected college men.' Los Angeles: Univ. So. Calif. Press. Quoted by Itkin

PATTERSON, C. H. 1943. 'The relationship of Bernreuter personality scores to other parent characteristics.' *J. Soc. Psych.*, **17,** 77–88.

PECK, R. F. and HAVIGHURST, R. J. 1960. *The Psychology of Character Development.* New York: Wiley

PIAGET, J. 1926. *La representation du monde chez l'enfant.* Paris.

PIAGET, J. 1932. *The moral judgement of the child.* London: Kegan Paul

PAIGET, J. 1968. *The Moral Judgement of the Child.* J. Piaget with the assistance of seven collaborators. Trans. from the French by Majorie Gabain. London: Routledge & Kegan Paul

POLLITT, J. 1967. *Depression and its Treatment.* London: Heinemann

POWER, M. 1966. *Families before the Courts.* Annual Review of the Residential Child Care Assoc.

QUAY, H. C. 1965. *Juvenile Delinquency.* New York: Van Nostrand Co.

RADKE, M. J. 1946. *The Relation Of Parental Authority To Children's Behaviour And Attitudes.* Univ. Minnesota Press

READ, K. H. 1945. 'Parents' expressed attitudes and children's behaviour.' *J. Consult. Psych.*, **9,** 95–100

REICH, W. 1925. *Der Triebhafte Charakter.* Vienna

RIEMER, M. D. 1940. 'Runaway Children.' *Amer. J. Ortho. Psychiat.*, **10,** 522

ROSE, D. E. 1949. 'Social Factors in delinquency.' *Aust. J. Psych.*, **1,** No. 1, 1

ROSE, G. N. G. 1968. 'The Artificial Delinquent Generation'. *J. Criminal Law, Criminal & Pol. Sci.* **59**(3), Sept., 370–85

ROSENHEIM, F. 1942. 'Character study of a rejected child.' *Amer. J. Ortho. Psychiat.*, **12,** 487

RUTTER, M. 1966. *Children of Sick Parents*, an environmental and psychiatric study. (Inst. of Psychiatry Maudsley Monograph, No. 16). Oxford University Press

SARBIN, T. R. and MILLER, J. E. 1970. 'Demonism Revisited: The XYY Chromosomal Anomaly'. *In Issues in Criminology*, **5,** no. 2, 195–207

SARGANT, W. 1957. *Battle for the Mind.* London: Heinemann

SARGANT, W. and SLATER, P. 1964. *Introduction to Physical Methods of Treatment in Psychiatry.* Edinburgh: Livingstone

SCHACTER, S. 1961. *The Psychology of Affiliation.* London: Tavistock Publications

SCHAEFER, E. S. 1959. 'A Circumplex Model for Maternal Behaviour'. *J. Abnorm. Soc. Psychol.* **59**, 226–236

SECORD, P. F. and BACKMAN, C. W. 1964. *Social Psychology.* New York: McGraw-Hill

SELLIN, T. and WOLFGANG, M. E. 1964. *The Measurement of Delinquency.* New York: Wiley

SEWALL, N. 1930. 'Some causes of jealousy in young children.' Smith Coll. Stud. Soc. Wk., **1**, 16–22. Quoted by Shoben

SHAW, C. R. 1929. *Delinquency Areas.* Univ. Chicago Press

SHAW, C. R. 1938. *Brothers in Crime.* Univ. Chicago Press

SHAW, C. R. and MCKAY, H. D. 1931. Social Factors in Juvenile Delinquency. Wash. (Nat. Comm. on Law Observance and Enforcement. Report on Causes of Crime, 2, No. 13).

SHAW, C. R., MCKAY, H. D. and MCDONALD, J. F. 1942. *Juvenile Delinquency in Urban Areas.* Univ. Chicago Press

SHIELDS, J. 1962. *Monozygotic Twins.* Oxford University Press

SHIELDS, R. W. 1962. *A Cure of Delinquents.* London: Heinemann

SHOBENE, E. J. 1949. 'The assessment of parental attitudes in relation to child adjustment.' *Genet. Psychol. Monogr.,* **39**, 101–148

SILVERMAN, B. 1935. 'The behaviour of children from broken homes.' *Amer. J. Ortho. Psychiat.,* **5**, 11

SILVERMAN, B. 1937. *J. Exp. Educ.,* **6**, 187

SIMPSON, M. 1935. *Parent Preferences of Young Children.* New York: Teachers Coll., Columbia Univ. Quoted by Itkin

SLAVSON, S. R. 1943. 'Treatment of aggression through group therapy.' *Amer. J. Ortho. Psychiat.,* **13**, 419

SLAVSON, S. R. 1965. *Reclaiming the Delinquent by Para-Analytic Group Psychotherapy in the Inversion Technique.* New York. Free P., Collier-Macmillan

SPROTT, W. J. H. 1952. *Social Psychology.* London: Methuen

STEKEL, W. 1925. *Peculiarities of Behaviour.* London: Williams and Norgate

STOGDILL, R. M. 1933. 'Attitude of parents, students, and mental hygienists towards children's behaviour.' *J. Soc. Psych.,* **4**, 486–489

STOGDILL, R. M. 1936. 'Experiments in the measurements of attitudes towards children: 1899–1936.' *Child Develop.,* **7**, 31–36. Quoted by Itkin

STOTT, D. H. 1950. *Delinquency and Human Nature.* Dunfermline Carnegie Trust

STOTT, L. H. 1940. 'Adolescents' dislikes regarding parental behaviour and their significance.' *J. Genet. Psycho.,* **57**, 393–414

STOTT, L. H. 1940(a). 'Parental attitudes of farm, town, and city parents in relation to certain personality adjustments in their children.' *J. Soc. Psycho.,* **11**, 325–339

SULLIVAN, C. E., GRANT, M. Q. and GRANT, J. D. 1954. *Delinquency Integrations: 2nd technical report.*
Article prepared for Neuro-psychiatric Brand, Bureau of Medicine and Surgery, Corrective Service, San Francisco State Coll. Office of Naval Research

SYMONDS, P. M. 1939. *The Psychology of Parent-child Relationships.* New York: D. Appleton-Century

TENNENBAUM, R. 1939. *Jewish Parents in a Child Guidance Clinic: A study of culture and personality.* Smith Coll. Study Soc. Wk., **10**, 50–76. Quoted by Itkin

TRASLER, G. 1962. *The Explanation of Criminality.* London: Routledge & Kegan Paul

VERNON, P. 1964. *Personality Assessment.* London: Methuen

VERNON, P. 1969. *Intelligence and Cultural Environment.* London: Methuen

VENESS, T. 1962. *School Leavers: their aspirations and expectations.* London: Methuen

WALKER, N. 1965. *Crime and Punishment in Britain.* Edinburgh: Edinburgh University Press

WALKER, N. 1969. *Sentencing in a Rational Society.* London: Allen Lane

WATSON, G. 1933. A critical note on two attitude studies. *Ment. Hyg.* **17**, 59–64

WATZLAWICK, P., BEAVIN, J. M. and JACKSON, D. D. 1968. *Pragmatics of Human Communication.* London: Faber & Faber

WEST, D. 1967. *The Young Offender.* London: Duckworth

WEST, D. 1969. *Present Conduct and Future Delinquency.* London: Heinemann

WHYTE, W. F. 1943. *Street Corner Society.* Univ. Chicago Press

WILKINS, L. T. 1964. *Social Deviance.* London: Tavistock Publications

WILKINS, L. 1964. *Delinquent Generations.* London: H.M.S.O.

WINNICOTT, D. W. 1958. *Collected Essays*

WINNICOTT, D. W. 1965. *The Family and Individual Development.* London: Tavistock Publications

WOLFGANG, M. E. and FERRACUTTI, F. 1967. *The Subculture of Violence.* London: Tavistock Publications

WOLLBERG, L. 1954. *The Techniques of Psychotherapy.* New York: Grune and Stratton

WOODWARD, M. 1955. *Low Intelligence and Delinquency.* Institute for the Study and Treatment of Delinquency

WOOTTON, B. 1959. *Social Science and Social Pathology.* London: Allen & Unwin

YARROW, M. R., LEEUW, L. and SCOTT, P. 1962. 'Child Rearing in Families of Working and Non-Working Mothers'. *Sociometry.* **25**, 122–140

YARROW, M. R. and GOODWIN, M. S. 1963. 'Effects of Change in Mother Figure during Infancy on Personality Development'. Progress Report *Family and Child Services*, Washington D.C.

ZILBOORG, G. 1937. 'Consideration of suicide with particular reference to that of the young.' *Amer. J. Ortho. Psychiat.*, **7**, 15

ZIMMERMAN, O. see Symonds
ZUCKER, H. 1943. 'The emotional attachment of children to their parents as related to standards of behaviour and delinquency.' *J. Psychol*, **15**, 31–40

3 : INTERVIEW-QUESTIONNAIRE

FOR YOUR INFORMATION ABOUT THIS INTERVIEW

People have different ideas about many things in different countries.

You are being interviewed in order to find out how differently people think in England, for instance, as compared with people in such faraway countries as Australia.

Your answer will be treated as *strictly confidential*.

Your *full co-operation* will be greatly appreciated in the interest of this research programme.

SURNAME	Christian Name(s)	Date of Birth	Age	Address
....	....	....	.... ..	....
	....		.. ;	....
	....		..	....

I.Q. ....   EDUCATION RETARDATION: Yes.... No....

OFFENCES:

No. of offence	Type of charges	Accomplices or not?	Was boy leader or not?	Date and age	Court	Remand or custody	Action
1st Offence							
2nd Offence							
3rd Offence							

N.B. (1) The questionnaire has been phrased to be addressed to the boy, hence requires appropriate rephrasing when used for parents.

(2) Answers to be scored as follows:
(*a*) answer of the boy to be scored with black pencil,
(*b*) answer of the mother to be scored with red pencil,
(*c*) answer of the father to be scored with blue pencil.

FAVOURITISM OF SIBLINGS

Ask all boys

1.1 Please tell me the names of your ....
brothers and sisters in the order in ....
which they were born.   ....

1.2 Who do you think is mother's
favourite? ....
And who comes next? ....
and next? ....
and next? ....
and after that? ....

1.3 Who do you think is father's favourite?
....
And who comes next? ....
and next? ....
and next? ....
and after that? ....

Names of siblings	Ranking	
	Mother's favourites	Father's favourites

Ask all parents

1.4 Please tell me the names of your ....
     children in the order in which they ....
     were born.   ....

1.5 Which is your favourite?   .:......................
                   And who comes next? ....
                             and next? ....
                             and next? ....
                         and after that? ....

PARENTAL WORK RECORD

Mother

2.1 Is mother working at present – or Yes........   No........
     has she done so up to the last few ....
     weeks.

2.1 What sort of work does mother ....
     do?   ....
     Is it full-time or part-time? Full-time....Part-time....

2.3 How old were you when your
     mother first started to go out to
     work?   ....

2.4 At what time does your mother
     come home after work?   ....

Father

2.4 What is your father's job?   ....

2.5 What jobs did he have before this
     one?   ....

2.6 Is your father very often on shift Shift work ....
     work, or on overtime work, or on Overtime work ....
     work that takes him away from Away from home ....
     home overnight?   ....

2.7 How old were you when your
     father was frequently on shift work
     or away?   ....

INFORMATION CONCERNING GRANDPARENTS

Father

3.1 Are father's parents still alive?   ....

If not, when did father's father

die?   P.F:....................

father's mother die? P.M: ....

3.2 Did father's parents live apart? Y........... N.........

3.3 Who moved out (or died)?   F......... M.........

3.4 When was this?   ....

AGE: ....

3.5 What was the reason? Please ....

state: ....

3.6 If at all, when was a reconciliation

affected?   ....

AGE: ....

3.7 What separations occurred be- ....

tween you and your parents? ....

Details: ....

3.8 Father's occupation: ....

Mother

3.9 Are mother's parents still alive?   ....

If not, when did mother's mother

die?   M.M. ....

mother's father die? M.F. ....

3.10 Did mother's parents live apart? Y......... N. ....

3.11 Who moved out (or died)?   F......... M. ....

3.12 When was this?   ....

AGE: ....

3.13 What was the reason? Please

state   ....

3.14 If at all, when was a reconciliation

affected?   ....

AGE: ....

3.15 What separations occurred between you and your parents?
Details: . . . .

3.16 Father's occupation: . . . .

DETAILS REGARDING DELINQUENCY

4.1 How old were you when you first
truanted? AGE: . . . .

4.2 Tell me all about this . . . .
. . . .

4.3 How old were you when you first
started to 'take things' that did not
belong to you? AGE: . . . .

4.4 Tell me what happened . . . .

4.5 Tell me about your present trouble . . . .

4.6 Has your mother become stricter More:
since you first got into trouble? Less:
Same:

4.7 Has your father become stricter More:
since you first got into trouble? Less:
Same:

PHYSICAL SEPARATIONS

5.1 Have you had any illnesses which
made it necessary for you to go to
hospital for more than a week during the first three years of your
life? . . . .
How old were you, what was the illness, how long did it last,
how long were you in hospital?

Age	Kind of illness	How long did it last?	Hospital?	If so, how long for?
1.				
2.				
3.				

5.2 Were you evacuated on your own– ....
that is, sent away because of the
bombing during the war?   YES   NO

5.3 How old were you at the beginning
and at the end of this evacuation? From   to
Age: ...... Age: ......

5.4 Were you evacuated with your
mother during the war?   ....

5.5 Who did you stay with during
evacuation?   ....

5.6 How did you like the people who
looked after you?   ....

5.7 How long has close contact lasted
for between you and these people? ....

5.8 What kind of contact, if any,
existed between you and your
parents at that time?

5.9 When you came back from
evacuation, do you think there
was less feeling for a while between: i. you and your mother:
ii. you and your father?

5.10 Was your father away during the
war?

5.11 How old were you at the beginning
and at the end of his war
service?

5.12 Were there any other separations,
apart from evacuation and your
illnesses, between you and either
of your parents? (e.g. has your
mother or your father been ill and
had to go to hospital?)

INFANT TRAINING

(Mother to be regarded as major informant Qs.6.1 – 6.11)

6.1 Was your boy breast-fed?   YES   NO

6.2 How old was he when breast-feeding stopped?   Aged: ....

6.3 Did you give him milk whenever he cried, or only at regular intervals?

whenever baby cried   at regular intervals

Normal   Retarded   Advanced ?

6.4 Was your boy's bowel training .. ..

6.5 Was your boy's bladder training .. ..

6.6 Sitting up .. .. ..

7.6 Cutting teeth .. ..

6.8 Walking .. .. ..

6.9 Talking .. .. ..

6.10 Was your boy a cross baby?   YES   NO

6.11 If cross, how old was he when he grew out of it?   Age: ....

THE CHILD AND SIBLINGS

7.1 If at all, with which brother or sister do you seem to quarrel mostly?

7.2 Which brother or sister do you seem to like best?

AFFECTION

(a) *Some details re attitudes and beliefs:*

	Both	Mother's family	Father's family	Nr.
8.1 Do you think that you look more like your mother (or her family) or like your father (or his family)?				

	Mother's	*Father's*	
Both	*family*	*family*	*Nr.*

8.2　In which way?

8.3　Whose ways do you have–
　　　Your mother's
　　　or your father's

8.4　In which way?

8.5　Which parent is more inclined
　　　to stick up for you even
　　　though you may be in the
　　　wrong?

8.6　Has this always been so?　　　YES　　　　NO

8.7　If not always, since when?

Special *note of information:* Please remember that answers to the following questions are very personal ones and therefore *strictly confidential.*

Answers can usually be given after some very deep and secret thinking. Please try to help to answer these questions to the best of your ability.

(b) Demonstration of affection

							What
M.	*F.*	*B.*	*Nr.*	*?*	*N.A.*		*else*

8.8　Is your mother
　　　the kind of per-
　　　son who gets
　　　rather embarras-
　　　sed to show
　　　openly that she　*A.*　　*B.*
　　　loves you?　　Y N?　Y N?

8.9　Is father ditto? Y N?　Y N?

8.10 Are you　ditto? Y N?　Y N?

8.11 Which　parent　gets　more
　　　embarrassed　to　show　love
　　　openly?

(*c*) *Affect* (For your special attention)

8.12 Which parent may honestly love you secretly a *little* more (or feel kindness more easily towards you, or have slightly closer bonds of affection with you, or feel closer to you)?

(*d*) *Over-sufficiency of affect*

8.13 Which parent do you think loves you perhaps just a little too much than may be good for you?

(*e*) *Under-sufficiency of affect*

8.14 Which parent may give *too little love*, affection and kindness to you?

(*f*) *Sufficiency of affect*

8.15 Which one of your parents is probably the one that gives the EXACT amount of affection to you?

(*g*) *Future*

8.16 Who should love you more in the *future*?

(*h*) *Whose favourite?*

8.17 Are you mother's boy or father's boy?

Ask 8.18 *of Mother only*

8.18 Were you your mother's girl or your father's girl?

Ask 8.19 *of Father only*

8.19 Were you your mother's boy or your father's boy?

What

M. F. B. Nr. ? N.A. *else*

(*i*) *Naggging*

8.20 If at all, which parent is more
inclined to 'nag' a lot (e.g.
complains often)?

8.21 If at all, which parent is inclined to pick on you?

HOME CLIMATE

9.1 Do your parents often quarrel in
front of you?   YES   NO

9.2 Do your parents quarrel slightly
more than average parents?   YES   NO

9.3 Which parent is usually more
cheerful at home?

TRAINING (PUNISHMENT, ETC.)

M.   F.   Nr.   ?   *What*
else

10.1 Which parent has, in fact, the final
say in your home, i.e. is the boss?

10.2 Which parent mostly punishes
you?

10.3 Which parent is slightly stricter at
home?

10.4 Which parent is rather too strict at
home?

10.5 Which parent is rather too lenient
at home?

10.6 Which parent is JUST RIGHT
regarding strictness at home?

10.7 Which parent often threatens with
punishment but never quite carries
it out in the end?

10.8 Which parent usually carries out punishment after a previous warn ing has been given?

10.9 Which parent should be stricter in your home in the future?

10.10 Which parent do you usually obey at home?

10.11 Why is this so? regarding obeying?

10.12 What kind of punishment works best with you?

10.13 Which parent praises you more often when you have done something well?

10.14 Which parent should in future praise you more often when you have done something well?

10.15 Which parent is rather too quick-tempered and flares up when he/she hears of trouble?

10.16 Which parent usually keeps cool and reasonable during trouble? (If neither, say so!)

10.17 Which parent *keeps it up* far too long after the trouble has been dealt with (doesn't forgive)?

10.18 Which parent *does not keep it up* long enough after the trouble has been dealt with (forgives too quickly)?

PSYCHOLOGICAL COMMUNICATION

M.   F.   B.   Nr.   N.A.   ?

11.1 Which parent actually knows more
about you?

11.2 Are you inclined to consult your
parents when in trouble? (Or do
you try to wriggle out of it?)   YES   NO   ?

M.   F.   B.   Nr.   N.A.   ?

11.3 Which parent do you usually go to
at first when you have done something wrong?

11.4 Why this parent at first?

11.5 Which parent do you prefer eventually and finally to 'deal with
your case' if you have done something wrong?

11.6 Why this parent eventually?

11.7 Which parent do you go to *at first*
when you want some advice?

DYNAMICS

(a) General Stress Reactions

12.1 When you seem to come up against
something you do not like – how
do you react or what do you do   *Troubles*
then?   *Major*   *Minor*
e.g. (i) Do you get rather nasty?
(ii) Do you become very
'sulky' or withdrawn?
(iii) Do you try to forget about
it quickly?
(iv) Or what else do you do?

12.2 How soon do you 'get over it'?   *Q*   *N.Q.*
Quickly or not?

M.   F.   B.   Nr.   N.A.   ?

12.3 Which parent are you more like in
this way?

(b) Specific Reaction to Parents:

12.4 How much do you seem to resent   *Resentful*   *Not Resentful*
     punishment from your parents?   Open   Secretly

(c) General Sociability

12.5 Do you prefer to play with other
     children or to keep to yourself?   YES   NO   ?

12.6 What do you do when you are out-
     of-doors?

12.7 Do you attend Sunday School or
     Church or Church-Club?   YES   NO   ?

Environmental Communication

13.1 Does your father often take you to
     outings, such as football games,
     etc. (compared with average
     fathers)?   YES   NO   ?

13.2 Should you do this sort of thing? YES   NO   ?

13.3 If he does not, why not?

13.4 Would it be helpful if your father
     saw a good deal more of you in
     the future?   YES   NO   N.A.

13.5 Would it be helpful if your
     mother saw a good deal more of
     you in the future?   YES   NO   N.A.

13.6 Do you and your father share YES   NO   N.A.
     many hobbies together?   A   occasionally   Hardly
                                 lot   ever

13.7 What hobbies do you and your
     father share?

13.8 What kind of activities during
     leisure time do you and your
     mother share a lot?

13.9 Do you prefer to be 'indoors' at
     night?   IN   OUT

13.10 How many days a week are you
     'indoors' at night?   DAYS

13.11 With whom do you spend most of
     your time when 'indoors'? Name:

                                   Age:..........

13.12 With which parent do you spend
     a bit more leisure time at night? *M. F. B. Nr. N.A. ?*

13.13 How much time do you and your Slightly more Sl. less Av.
     father spend together during than average   av.
     week-ends?

13.14 How much time do you and your
     mother spend together during
     week-ends?

13.15 State what you do usually on
     Sundays?

Other Information:

14.1 Finally any other important in-
     formation to be discussed in this
     'Questionnaire-Interview'?

INDEX

Note: Index does not cover Appendices 1 and 2. For each subject (but not author) reference, the major pages have been given bold face numerals.

187